Postpartum Nutrition

An Expert's Guide to Eating After a Baby

ISBN 978-1-8382509-1-1

This book is sold with the understanding that the author and publisher are not engaged in rendering medical, health or any other kind of personal professional services in the book. The reader should consult their own competent professional before adopting any of the suggestion in this book.

Postpartum and Beyond
EAT FOR HEALTH

Foreword by General Practitioner Dr Preeya Alexander

As a mother and general practitioner, I know how tricky the postpartum period can be. Knowing what to eat and how to support the body in the postpartum period can be very difficult particularly when new mothers are swamped with information and exhausted juggling their new child's needs with their own.

Harriet has beautifully broken down what the body (both mum and baby's) needs in the postpartum period. She gives you the nuts and bolts so you can make informed choices when it comes to diet and food choices.

I connected with Harriet on Instagram and have always admired the way she breaks down complex information around nutrition and medicine to give people bite-sized easy to digest information.

I wish I had read this before doing the postpartum journey all over again quite recently. Whilst I know some of it, having what the body needs broken down in a clear and concise manner reminds the exhausted "mum brain" how to best support the body when it comes to nutrition.

This is a really helpful guide for mothers – I just wish I had read it sooner!

Preeya

Dr Preeya Alexander MBBS FRACGP

HEALTHY EATING DR

fact not fiction

contents

HEALTHY EATING DR

fact not fiction

contents

Postpartum and Beyond

EAT FOR HEALTH

Introduction

Firstly, congratulations on your new baby! This is an exciting time for you and your family.

For many women, pregnancy can be a time which focuses their mind on what they are eating, but in the whirlwind of having a new baby, this can be forgotten. Eating well while breastfeeding can be really challenging with a new-born to take care of and a shortage of sleep. Even more so if you have an active toddler to contend with during the day as well. Latest evidence supports that you need higher levels of some micronutrients while breastfeeding to support your own long-term health. With so much conflicting information available online, it can also be difficult to sift the fact from fiction.

If you are searching for credible information, look no further as this book is just for you. The information is based on the latest guidance and scientific evidence.

I've included micronutrient weights and quantities in this book, not to scare you, or to encourage you to weigh your food, but to give you some confidence and reassurance that on an average week you are eating enough. Without these quantities, it can be hard to tell.

Also included is a section introducing the essentials of weaning, and how to wean your baby onto a vegetarian or vegan diet. Unsure which vitamins your baby needs and when? There is information on vitamins for children depending on their age, and if they drink formula milk. Cow's milk protein allergy can be a struggle for parents, so I've included information about what it is, the latest guidance and how to choose a dairy free / plant based milk.

Introduction continued...

Your body has been through a huge change during pregnancy and post birth. Many women get frustrated that they don't just 'bounce back' like some celebrities do. Instead you might want to have more information about how and when to start thinking about getting back to a healthy weight.

About Me

I studied medicine at the University of Cambridge and have over a decade of experience as a paediatric doctor. Additionally I have a PhD in genetics from University College London. I am a Registered Nutritionist with the Association for Nutrition and was commissioned to write the first degree of it's kind combining culinary, nutrition and health.

I now use these uniquely developed skills for the benefit of my clients and students, consulting as a Registered Nutritionist and lecturing in culinary science and nutrition. My focus is science backed nutrition. Follow me @healthyeatingdr for more nutrition facts not fiction, so that you can eat for health today.

Harriet x

Dr Harriet Holme MA Hons Cantab MBBS MRCPCH(2009) PhD RNutr

Postpartum and Beyond
EAT FOR HEALTH

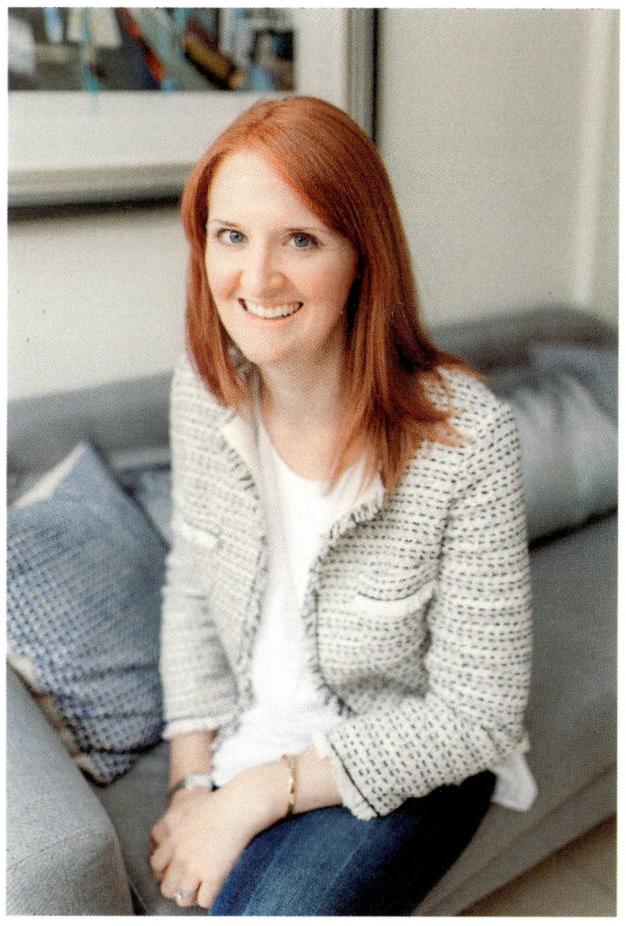

Dr Harriet Holme MA Hons Cantab MBBS MRCPCH(2009) PhD RNutr

Postpartum and Beyond

EAT FOR HEALTH

Guide to Eating Well After Birth

Eating well can be really challenging with a new-born to take care of and a shortage of sleep. Even more so if you have an active toddler to contend with during the day as well. Making sure that you are eating well can help your energy levels too. If you are breastfeeding, you only need approximately 400-500 extra calories each day, but you do need some additional micronutrients to protect your long term health.

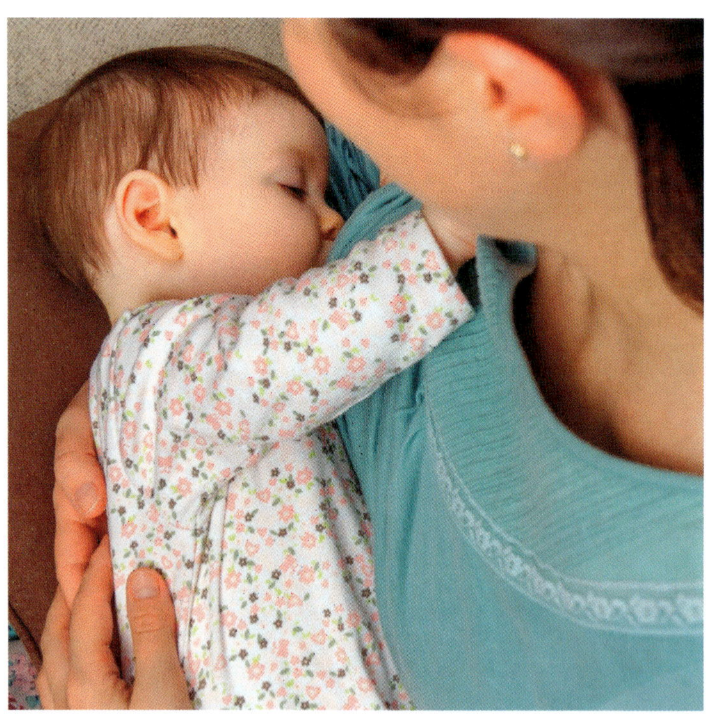

Postpartum and Beyond

EAT FOR HEALTH

Guide to Eating Well After Birth...

For breastfeeding mums of babies with allergies, having a diet with restrictions can be a barrier to getting enough of the nutrients you need, and you need to be more mindful of what you are eating. This is especially important for mums who need to exclude dairy and / or eggs. Both my children had Cow's Milk Protein Allergy (CMPA), and in the 2.5 years between them, I saw an explosion of dairy free products on the market and every local coffee shop had plant based milk. Restaurants now need allergen menus, so it is easier to eat out, with lots of supermarkets even having their own plant based milks. See below for my tips on how to ensure you are meeting your micronutrient needs.

In those early days of postpartum haze, smoothies can also be a great way of getting calories and nutrients in quickly, and are better than juices, as they contain more of the soluble and insoluble fibre which is so good for your gut.

Batch cooking can be a good way of filling your fridge and freezer with lots of nutritious meals that are ready to reheat. Lots of mums find they are especially hungry while breastfeeding, and so it's a good idea to have lots of healthy snacks to hand, for when temptation strikes!

Postpartum and Beyond
EAT FOR HEALTH

Guide to Eating Well After Birth...

Whatever your stage in life, there are some guiding principles for eating well. Think of foods to enjoy and those to swap out:

Enjoy:

- a wide range of colourful fruit and vegetables (aim for at least 5 a day)
- 2 portions of protein per day such as lean meat or fish, eggs, lentils, pulses, beans, and tofu etc, which are also an important source of iron.
- 3 portions of calcium rich food per day such as dairy products, or tinned fish, where you eat the bones, tahini, broccoli, tofu, almonds and dried fruit
- plenty of fluid (approximately 8 glasses), which is especially important in pregnancy as your blood supply increases
- eating with friends and family
- aim for a fibre intake of 30g (especially important immediately after giving birth) so enrich your diet with extra dried fruit, beans, and lentils, in addition to fruit, vegetables and whole grains.
- oily fish twice a week – why not have a regular fish night on Tuesday and Friday so it becomes part of your routine.
- a handful of nuts a day.

Postpartum and Beyond

EAT FOR HEALTH

Guide to Eating Well After Birth...

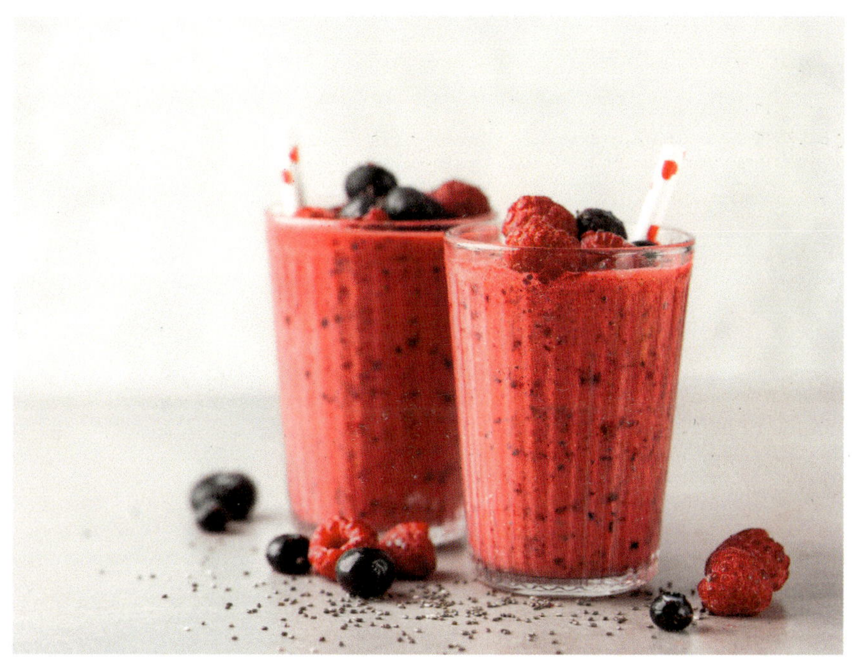

Guide to Eating Well After Birth

Swap out:

- refined carbohydrates for wholegrain
- carbohydrates (bulgur wheat, millet, brown bread, brown rice)
- sugary drinks for water
- saturated fats like butter, coconut and animal
- fat for lean protein and unsaturated fats such as avocado, extra virgin
- olive oil, and rapeseed oil.
- ready meals and added salt to home cooked whole foods.

In the next section, I discuss nutrient needs which vary according to whether you choose to breastfeed or not. Firstly are the micronutrients that all mums need in their diet, followed by calcium, iodine and selenium, needed in higher quantities for the long term health of breastfeeding mums.

Postpartum and Beyond
EAT FOR HEALTH

Guide to Eating Well After Birth

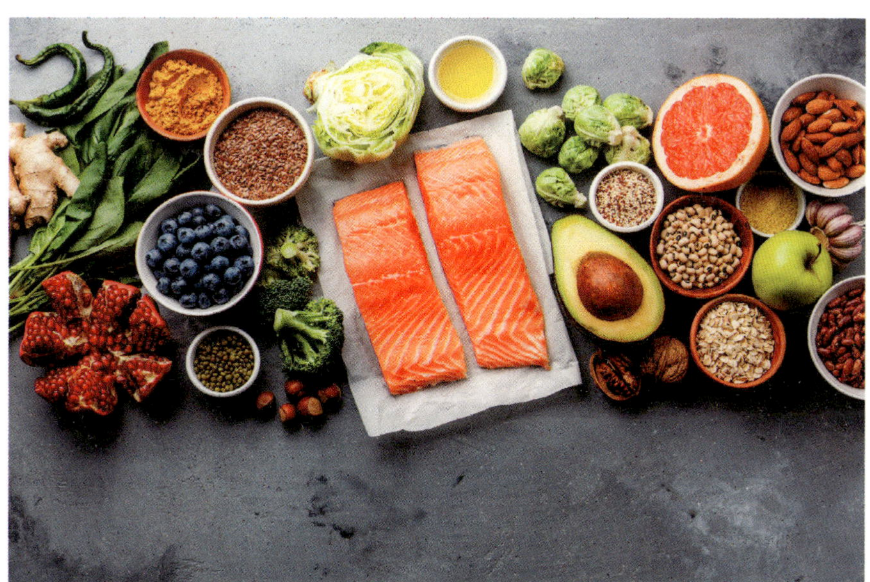

Vitamins and Minerals

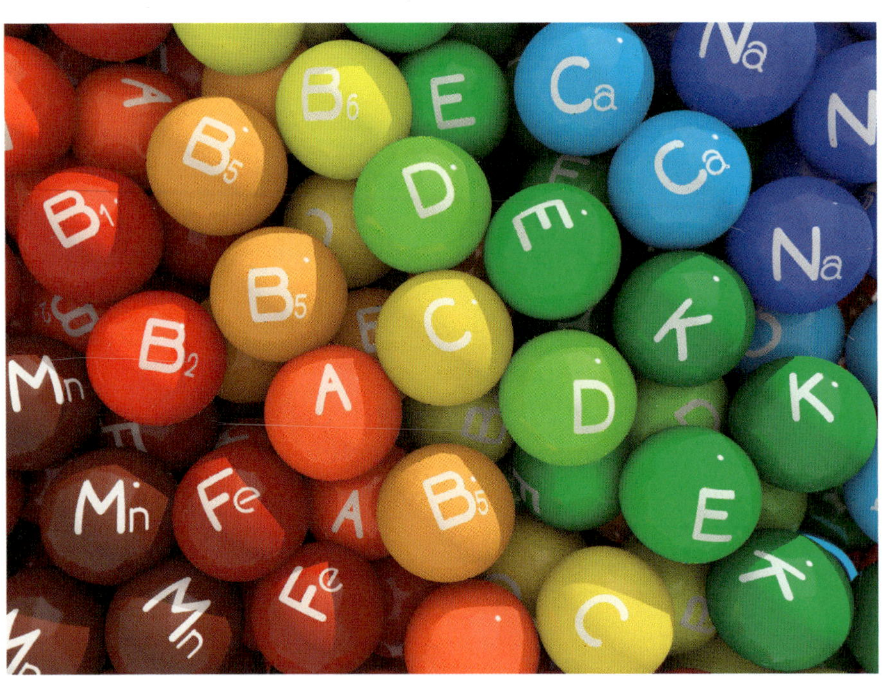

Vitamins and Minerals

Many people take a general pregnancy multi-vitamin during pregnancy and continue this during the postnatal period. However, there is no evidence of benefit of taking a general multi vitamin and mineral supplement unless you have specific health needs.

Instead there are key specific vitamins and minerals that are important alongside a balanced diet.

Vitamin D

Vitamin D is produced in your body using sunlight, and most people do not get enough without supplementing. It's recommended most people take a vitamin D supplement in the UK during autumn and winter.

Vitamin D is vital for optimal functioning of 20% of our genes and is produced using sunlight. Most people can't make enough from sunshine alone all year around in the UK. It's recommended most people take a vitamin D supplement during the autumn and winter. This is 10mcg or 400IU a day to maintain sufficient levels of vitamin D. Check what your local government recommendations are, as this will depend on your geographical location and how much sun you see.

Vitamin D plays an important role in calcium absorption from your gut, and together they both play a crucial role in bone health. For food combinations rich in vitamin D and calcium try:

- Scrambled eggs with spring greens such as kale
- Salmon and almonds

Iron

For most women there is no need to take an iron supplement unless you have had significant blood loss and are found to be anaemic. Instead you should be able to get your iron needs through your diet (dark green leafy vegetables, whole grains, tofu, beans, lentils and meat).

If however, you are found to be anaemic via a blood test, then your doctor will prescribe you an iron supplement.

Women between 19-50 years old need approximately 14.8mg of iron a day.

Some women are advised to take Spatone, as an iron supplement. This contains 5mg of iron per 25ml sachet and can be useful if your iron levels are borderline, or if you are struggling to include iron rich items in your diet.

The absorption of non-haem (plant based) iron is enhanced by vitamin C. Iron deficiency is common in both vegan and vegetarian diets, so this food combination may be helpful:

- Try any iron rich food such as broccoli, spinach, chickpeas and fruit such as blueberries for dessert.
- Lentils or bean salad, sprinkled with sunflower seeds and a lemon dressing

Caffeine can decrease absorption of plant based (non-haem) iron so avoid drinking a coffee or tea after your meal. Try herbal tea instead.

Iron

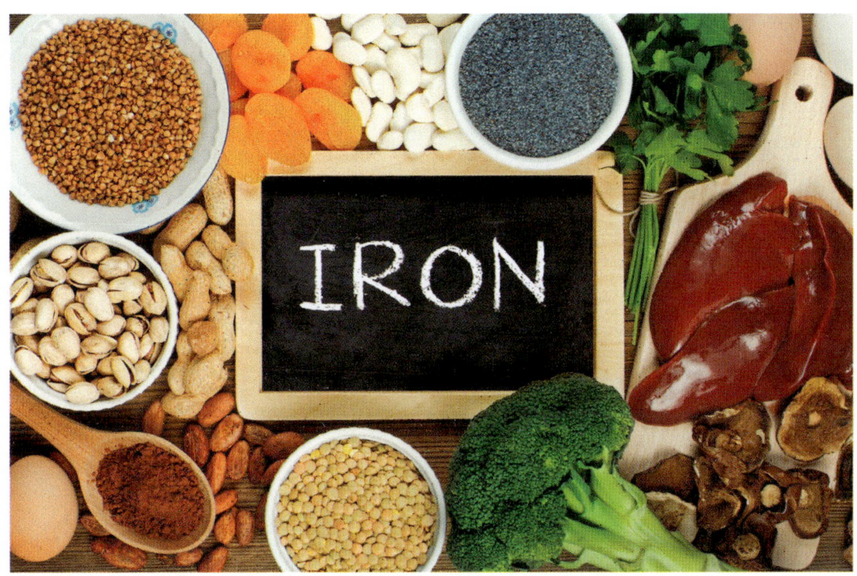

Iron...

Type of Food	Iron per 100g (mg)	Average portion size (g)	Iron per average portion size (mg)
Beef (rump steak)	3.6	100	3.6
Beef mince	2.7	90	2.4
Lamb leg	1.8	90	1.6
Chicken (light meat)	0.7	90	0.6
Liver pate	5.9	75	4.4
Pork Sausages	1.1	100	1.1
Egg	2.2	60	1.3
Cod / haddock	0.1	100	0.1
Salmon	0.4	100	0.4
Canned tuna	1.0	100	1
Baked beans in tomato sauce	1.4	100	1.4
Canned butter beans	1.5	100	1.5
Chickpeas	2.0	100	2
Kidney beans	2.0	100	2
Tofu	1.2	100	1.2
Figs (partially dried	3.9	50	2.0
Apricots (partially dried)	3.4	50	1.7
Dates	1.3	50	0.7
Brazil nuts	2.5	30	0.8
Smooth peanut butter	2.1	20	0.4
Hazelnuts	3.2	30	1.0
Sesame seeds	10.4	10	1.0
Sunflower seeds	6.4	15	1.0
Broccoli (boiled)	1.0	100	1
Spinach (boiled)	1.6	100	1.6

Source: https://www.bda.uk.com/resource/iron-rich-foods-iron-deficiency.html

Omega 3

Omega 3 fatty acids, are essential fats that can't be produced in your body and have to be eaten in your diet. It is found in a number of foods such as nuts, seeds and oily fish. The main types are eicosapentaenoic acid (EPA) and docosahexaenoi acid (DHA), both found in fish, and then alpha-linolenic acid (ALA) found in plant foods.

Omega 3 supplements often contain vitamin A, which should be avoided in pregnancy but there is no need to avoid them after you have had your baby.

Oily fish which is naturally high in omega 3 (see the guidance under the fish and shellfish section). The latest advice is to eat 1-2 portions a week. This is to balance the risk of contamination from heavy metals seen in larger fish at the top of the food chain.

If you are vegan, sources of ALA are seeds (chia, linseeds, and hemp), walnuts, soybeans, rapeseed oil, hazelnuts, pecans, green leafy vegetables and tofu.

While omega 3 was thought to benefit heart health, there is now strong evidence that omega-3 supplements do not seem to have the same heart health benefits as including oily fish in your diet, which may be related to the 'whole food effect' of oily fish.

Omega-3 may have a role in reducing the risk of certain cancers, treating arthritis, improving memory in older adults and treating depression, but further research in these areas is needed. If you are unable get enough omega fatty acids in your diet by eating foods rich in omega 3, then you might consider supplementing.

Omega 3

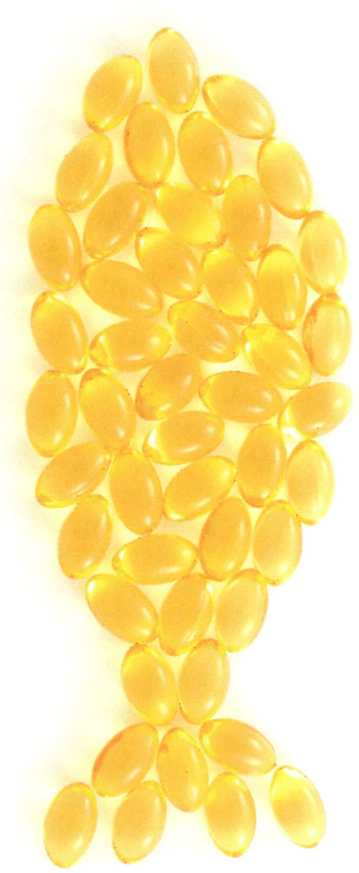

Your Nutrition While Breastfeeding

If you are breastfeeding it is recognised that there are some nutrients that you need more of to support your long term health. This is especially important if you exclude any food groups from your diet, such as dairy or eggs, as you might find it requires more planning to ensure you meet your micronutrient needs.

Calcium

Calcium is vital for bone health, and while that might not seem that relevant while you are young, remembering to look after your bones will help reduce your risk of fractures later in life. While you won't feel the immediate benefits of getting enough calcium today, in the future you will be grateful.

Women who are at highest risk of calcium deficiency are:

- vegan or dairy free
- have coeliac disease
- are breastfeeding
- past the menopause
- have osteoporosis (softening of the bones)

This means if you are breastfeeding and had to exclude dairy out of choice or because your baby has cow's milk protein allergy (CMPA), then you are at increased risk. When you choose a plant based milk, ensure that it has added calcium (see the plant based milk section).

Calcium...

If you are breastfeeding you need approximately 1250mg of calcium a day, while pre-menopausal women need 700mg a day, and women with Coeliac or Inflammatory bowel disease need 1000-1500mg per day.

Remember to include foods rich in calcium in your diet, either dairy products, or non-dairy such as tofu, pulses, dried fruit, and fish that have edible bones, such as sardines, or tinned salmon are a great source of calcium.

These are some examples of calcium rich food (that are also listed in the nutrient checklist at the end):

- 100mls of cow's milk (1/2 cup) = 125mg calcium
- 100ml fortified oat milk ~120mg
- 100ml fortified nut milks ~120mg
- 100ml The Mighty pea mylk ~186mg
- 100ml fortified coconut milk ~120mg
- matchbox size piece of cheese ~220mg
- 120mg yoghurt ~200mg
- 100mls (/2 cup) fortified orange juice ~120mg
- 1 slice calcium fortified bread ~190mg
- 1/2 tin sardines (with bones) ~260mg
- 50g (small portion) whitebait ~430mg
- 6 pieces of scampi (90g) ~190mg
- 2 slices wholemeal bread ~54mg
- 2 slices white bread ~100mg
- 1 pitta bread ~60mg
- 1 medium orange ~75mg
- 85mg boiled broccoli (2 spears) ~34mg
- 75mg spring greens ~55mg

Calcium...

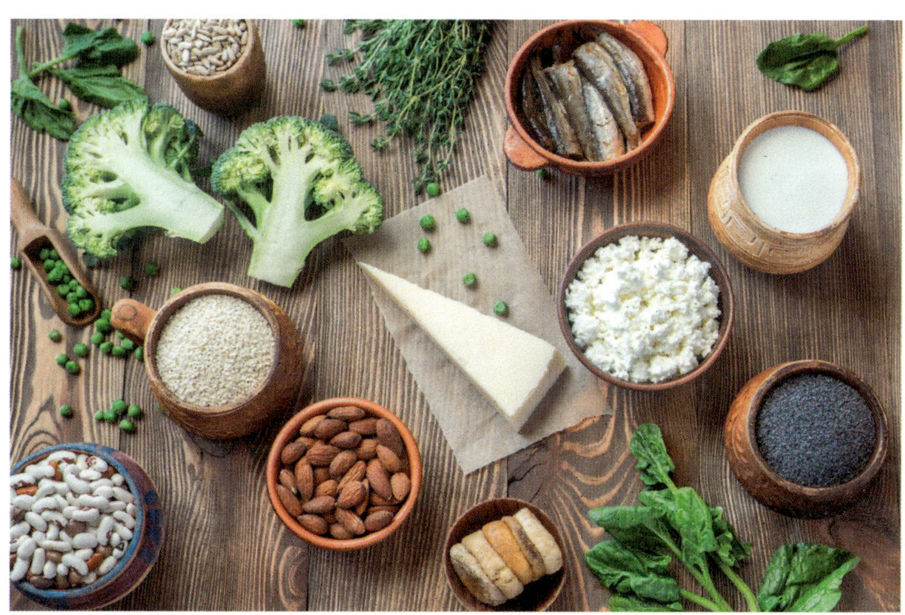

Calcium...

The calcium fortification in different brands will vary, so check the packaging to be sure.

As mentioned earlier, vitamin D plays an important role in calcium absorption from your gut, and together both play a crucial role in bone health. For food combinations rich in vitamin D and calcium try:

- Scrambled eggs with spring greens such as kale
- Salmon and almonds

There are concerns that calcium supplements might cause a sharp spike in the level of calcium in your blood, which is then at risk of being deposited in your blood vessels. If you are able to get enough calcium through your diet, this is preferable, but if not, your doctor may prescribe calcium supplements for you.

Exercise is really important for bone health and current guidance is to aim to walk, cycle, run, play tennis, Pilates or another sport for at least 30 minutes five times a week. Only consider this when you feel physically recovered from giving birth, and gradually introduce it back into your routine where possible.

You might find it initially impossible, but as a mother, once my children were walking, I found that I spent most of the day running around chasing after them! All exercise counts, it doesn't have to be formal.

Iodine

Iodine is another important micronutrient that until recently has been largely thought to be sufficient in our diets. However, research has raised concerns that pregnant and breastfeeding women are at risk of deficiency.

Dairy products and fish are iodine rich foods, so people following a vegan diet are at risk of iodine deficiency. If you are excluding dairy from your diet, a number of the plant based milks have just started to supplement with iodine as well as calcium, (see plant based milk section).

Depending on your life stage, people need different amounts of iodine per day:

- children 1-8 years need 90 mcg
- children 9-13 years need 120 mcg
- teenagers 14-18 years and adults need 150mcg
- pregnant and breastfeeding women need 200 mcg

To get 200mcg of iodine per day the following items would provide this but obviously you can mix and match from different sources to get your requirements:

- One portion of cod or haddock
- Or approximately 400-500mls of cow's milk
- Or 300-400g of dairy yoghurt
- Or 8 eggs
- Fortified plant milk (see plant milk section)

Iodine levels in food vary, and are higher in the winter.

Iodine

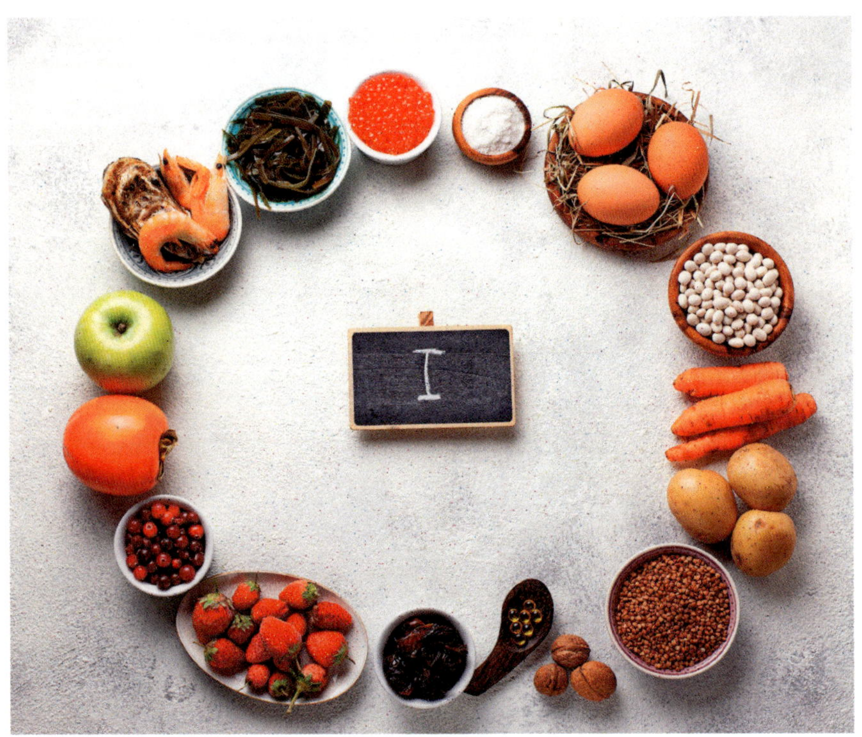

Selenium

Selenium is a micronutrient that doesn't often make the headlines, but it is important for your thyroid to work properly and fatigue can be a sign of deficiency. Breastfeeding mothers and pregnant women need the highest levels of 60 -70mcg per day. Foods rich in selenium are meat (organs more than muscles), fish, eggs and whole grains, but brazil nuts have a huge amount compared with other foods, with just one nut providing your daily requirement of selenium.

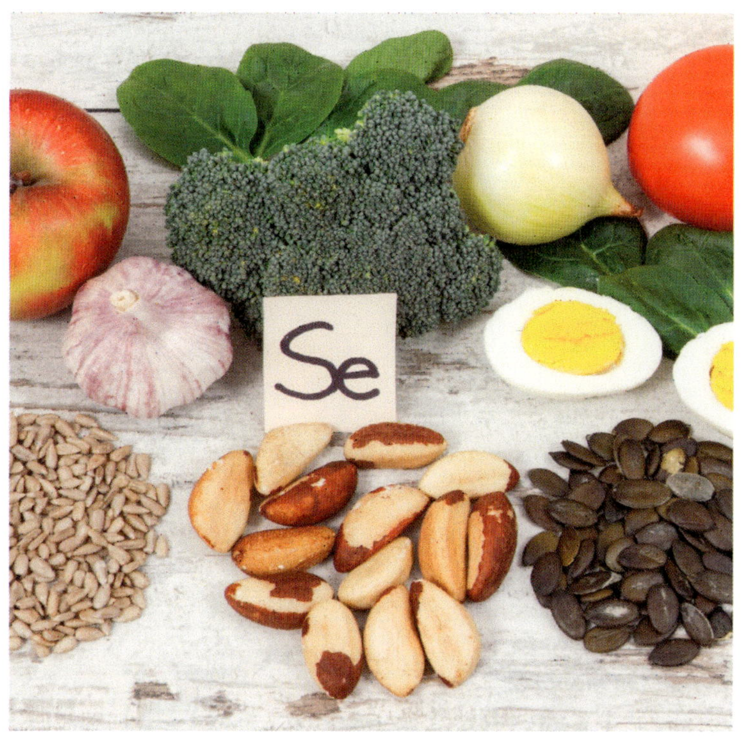

The Benefits of Breastmilk

As a mother of two children, I know from personal experience that breastfeeding can be tough and demanding but also very rewarding.

As a former paediatrician, I'm a strong advocate for mothers to be supported without judgement however they chose to feed their baby. Equally, I do think it is vitally important for mothers to have unbiased, science backed information so that they can make an informed choice about feeding.

There are a number of key reasons how breast milk is different to formula milk, and I'll talk through why this is important. Even more astonishingly, there is even a difference between pumped breast milk and direct transfer from the breast.

What is the microbiota?

While some bacteria are harmful, many are key to our health. The microbiota is the term used to cover the trillions of bugs, mostly made up of bacteria, that live on our skin and in our gut.

Why is the microbiota important?

We know that these single cell organisms play a huge role in many aspects of our health as adults, ranging from reduced risk of type 2 diabetes, obesity, immune function and even response to chemotherapy.

Postpartum and Beyond

EAT FOR HEALTH

The Benefits of Breastmilk

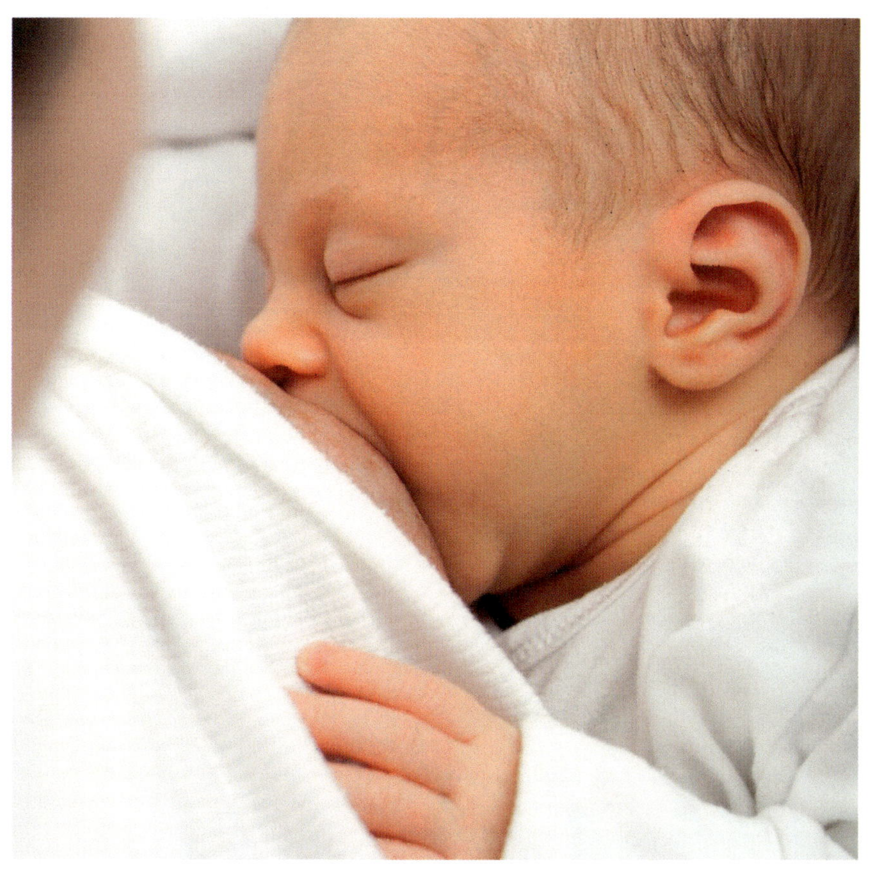

Postpartum and Beyond

EAT FOR HEALTH

The Benefits of Breastmilk...

When breastfeeding, the mother and baby although individuals, have an interactive relationship, that is called a dyad; this is highlighted by how the friendly microorganisms in breastmilk (milk microbiota) are formed. A healthy gut microbiota was first thought to be established by exposure through vaginal delivery and secondly through transfer of bacteria through breastmilk but there is now evidence that this is simplified, with many additional factors playing a role.

Live microorganisms are already found in breastmilk, even before a mother has breastfed her baby for the first time, providing evidence of maternal origin (called entero-mammary pathway). The microorganisms in the baby's mouth are similar to the mother's breastmilk. New evidence suggests that in addition to maternal transfer, there is also communication via the baby's saliva back into the breast, which also has a role in determining the microbiome.

Mode of delivery, older siblings, maternal and infant antibiotic exposure, complementary feeding with formula milk, and even mode of feeding (pumped breastmilk versus directly at the breast) are all thought to play a part in determining the baby's gut microbiome.

Some of these factors may only act in the short term, for example there is some evidence to suggest that mode of delivery has no persistent effect at 8 months. While others may have a more long term effect, for example, stool microbiome profiles of children at 1 year were significantly different in those that were still breastfed, compared to those that weren't. This was independent of previous antibiotic exposure or mode of delivery.

The Benefits of Breastmilk...

More research is still needed to determine why the microbiota is different with pumped breastmilk compared with direct transfer, to answer whether it is the act of pumping or lack of contact with the baby's mouth.

Ultimately whether breastmilk provides the microorganisms to colonise the baby's gut, or provides nutrients and prebiotics to foster a specific environment for selective growth of certain microorganisms, or a mixture of both, has yet to be fully established. However, maturation and maintenance of the lining of the infant gut depends on bacterial colonisation and with evidence to support a long-term health impact.

Is breastmilk different to formula milk?

Breastmilk contains a number of different components that make it different to formula milk, that are hard to replicate. In addition to the microorganisms, other components of breastmilk such as immune cells, fatty acids, antibodies, and human milk oligosaccharides (HMOs), also have a role in shaping the diversity of organisms.

Postpartum and Beyond

EAT FOR HEALTH

The Benefits of Breastmilk

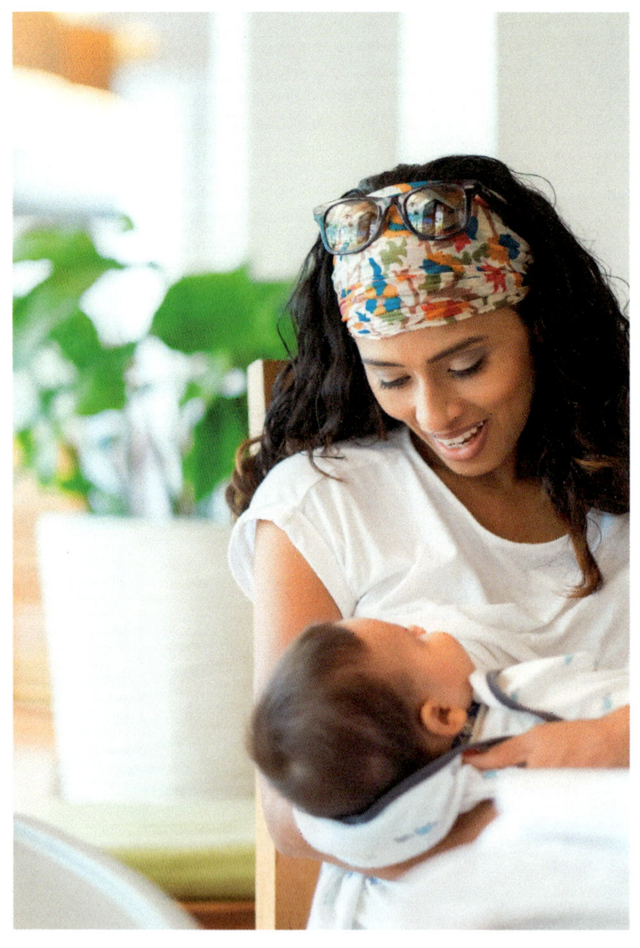

The Benefits of Breastmilk...

Human Milk Oligosaccharides

Human milk oligosaccharides (HMOs) are short chain carbohydrates, which are present in breastmilk that are essentially undigested by the baby, but are an important nutrient source for specific types of bacteria in the gut, called prebiotics. One of the bacteria commonly seen in the gut of healthy babies is Bifidobacterium longus infantis that metabolise HMOs into acetate and lactate.

These compounds are acidic, and change the pH of the infant stool, which are associated with lower levels of potentially harmful bacteria and those that harm the lining of the gut. The formation of other bacteria that are potentially harmful, maybe prevented by HMOs, thereby shaping the formation of the microbiota, improving the barrier function of the lining of the gut, and playing a role in immune function.

Lactoferrin

Lactoferrin, found in breastmilk, binds iron for transfer and aids it's absorption through the infant gut lining. This has a duel role, firstly helping the baby to absorb and use this iron as an important nutrient, and also leading to a reduction of the quantity of iron in the gut, which prevents harmful bacterial growth.

The Benefits of Breastmilk...

Antibodies in Breastmilk

Antibodies are used to tag microbes like viruses and bacteria, for destruction by other immune cells. Levels of certain antibodies (IgA, IgG and IgM), have been found to be higher in the guts of babies who are breastfeed. When babies are born, they are initially unable to produce the antibodies they need.

Breastmilk functions to supply these antibodies for the first few weeks until the baby is able to produce enough themselves. Supply of antibodies from breastmilk means that babies who are breastfed, have a lower risk of some childhood infections.

Low levels of antibodies (specifically IgA), as a baby has been associated with increased risk of development of allergies and asthma during childhood, and development of Crohn's disease (chronic inflammatory condition of the gut), in children.

Xanthine Oxidase

Interestingly breastmilk contains an enzyme called xanthine oxidase, while neonatal saliva contains the substrates for this enzyme (xanthine and hypoxanthine). When the enzyme mixes with these substrates in the mouth and intestinal tract of the baby, a chemical reaction occurs, releasing hydrogen peroxide. This is antibacterial, and regulates the growth of some bacteria, possibly with a role in creating the different microbiome seen in breastfed babies.

The Benefits of Breastmilk...

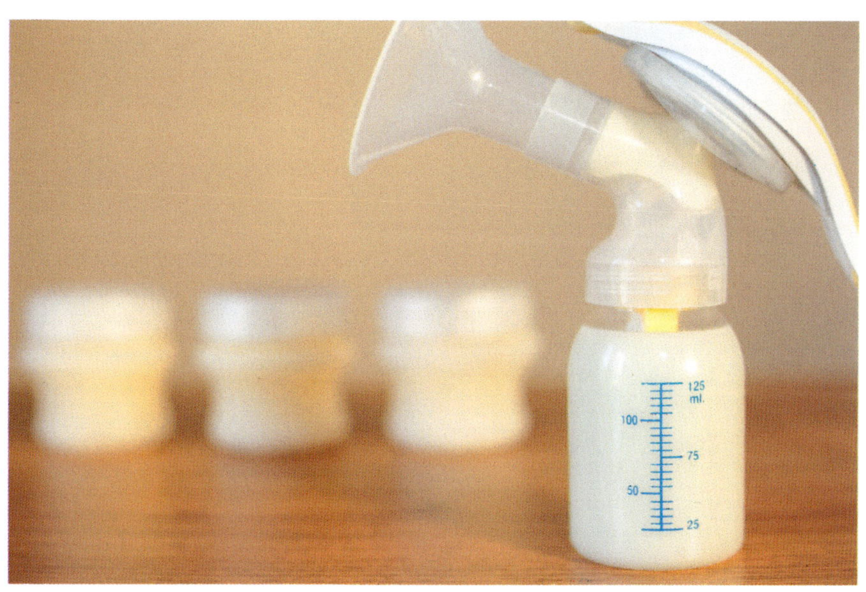

Postpartum and Beyond

EAT FOR HEALTH

The Benefits of Breastmilk...

Does the Type of Milk Matter?

Animal studies in monkeys have found that there are changes in the immune system in exclusively breastfed babies compared to those who are fed formula, and that these changes persist for 3-5 years after birth, long after weaning.

In humans, gut bacteria have been found to differ between exclusively breastfed and formula fed babies. Prebiotic like compounds added to formula milk, predict a microbiome distinct to that seen in an exclusively breastfed baby. While mixed fed babies have a microbiota that appears to be on a spectrum between that of breastfed and formula fed babies.

What about Weaning and the Microbiota?

Introduction of complementary foods (weaning) changes the microbiota in the baby's gut. Early weaning starting at 4 months or before, has been associated with a 30% higher risk of being overweight or obese (high Body Mass Index) in childhood, and a less diverse gut microbiota. A high Body Mass Index (BMI) in childhood is associated with a higher future risk of high cholesterol profile, high blood pressure, diabetes and cardiovascular disease.

However, those children who were breastfed for more than 4 months, did not have a higher BMI at 5 years, regardless of age at weaning, so breastfeeding appears to be protective.

The Benefits of Breastmilk...

Are there Benefits of Breastmilk Long Term?

The first 1000 days of life is a critical period for development of the immune system, and up to 70% is associated with the gut. In the first few months of life, patterns are established for recognising self and non-self (highly important in autoimmune diseases), that have life-long consequences.

There is evidence that the incidence of eczema, and wheezing in the first 2 years of life can be decreased by exclusive breastfeeding for 3 to 4 months. Additionally, evidence suggests that a longer duration of breastfeeding may protect against asthma after the age of 5 years. Breastfeeding has not been shown to prevent or delay the onset of specific food allergies.

Maternal Benefits of Breastfeeding

For mothers, in addition to the psychological aspect of bonding, breastfeeding decreases the risk of breast cancer and may protect against ovarian cancer and type 2 diabetes.

Postpartum and Beyond

EAT FOR HEALTH

The Benefits of Breastmilk

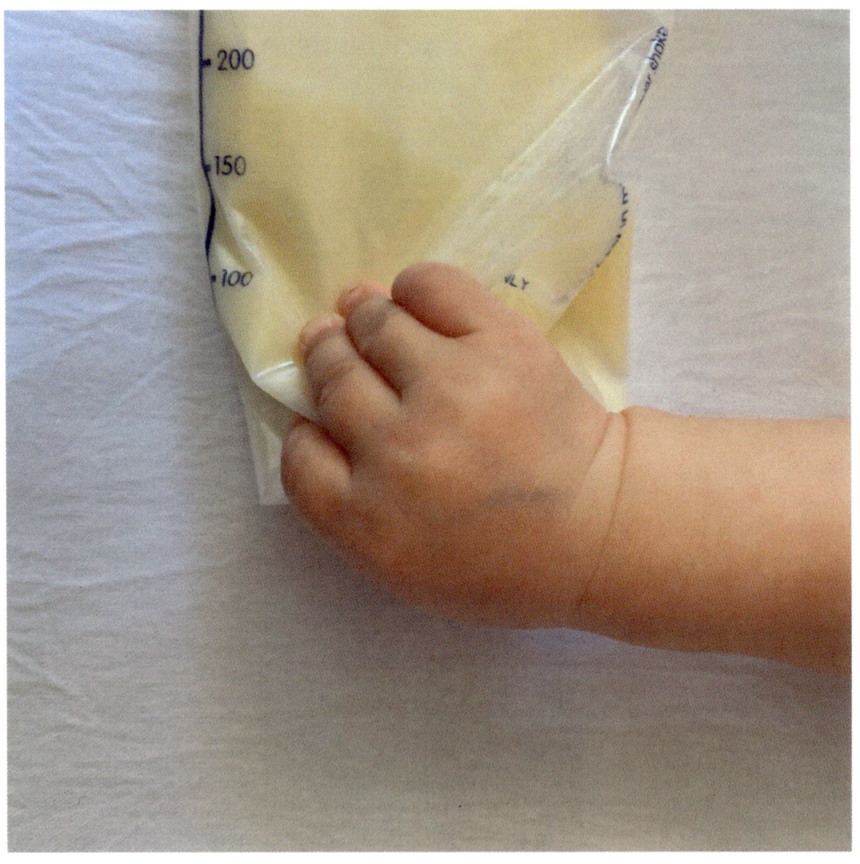

Drinking Alcohol While Breastfeeding

After 9 months of abstaining from alcohol, I think it's a question that many women want to know - can I drink alcohol and safely breastfeed my baby?

Limited drinking in moderation is safe for your baby but there are some simple tips to follow. While alcohol quickly enters your blood, it is also relatively quickly broken down and removed, at a rate of approximately 1 unit per hour. It can take up to an hour or longer if are eating food at the same time, before alcohol is present in your milk. So it's best to try to feed your baby before having an alcoholic drink and then there will naturally be a few hours before your baby is due their next feed.

'Pumping and dumping won't speed up elimination of alcohol and isn't needed if you plan ahead and time your drink to fit in with breastfeeding. If you plan to drink more and are concerned there won't be enough time for the alcohol to have been broken down, then you could use expressed milk for the next feed, pump for comfort (and to maintain your milk supply) and then return to breastfeeding.

It isn't recommended to drink alcohol at all for the first month or so. As with any alcohol advice, drink in moderation, avoid binges, aim for two alcohol free days a week, and have a maximum of 14 units per week.

If you have had any alcohol, you should avoid sharing a bed or sofa with your baby, as this has a strong association with sudden infant death syndrome.

Drinking Alcohol While Breastfeeding...

Alcohol is associated with increased risk of cancer, especially breast cancer, obesity, type 2 diabetes, cardiovascular disease and liver disease. These risks are higher if you drink more than 14 units per week.

There is no 'safe' drinking level, but drinking less than 14 units a week is considered low risk drinking. There is limited evidence that drinking red wine, since it contains more polyphenol compounds (natural antioxidants) may be a better choice than a spirt.

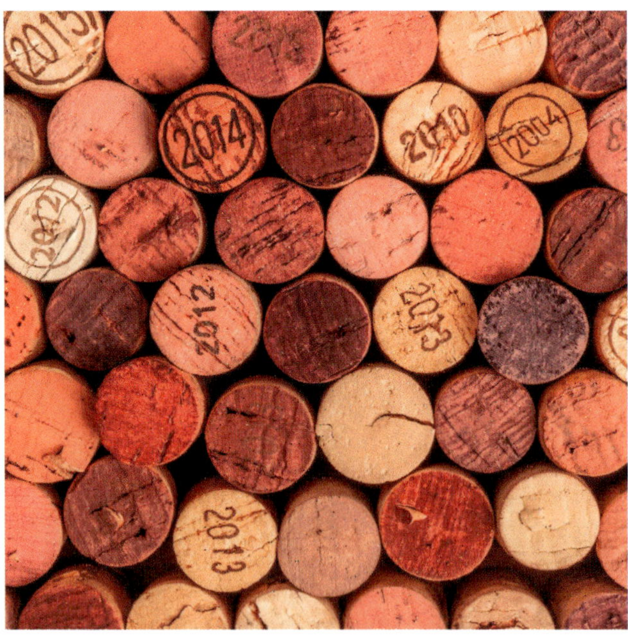

Cow's Milk Protein Allergy and Reflux

Both my babies had CMPA, and it was a difficult time for us as a family. Not only did we have the usual sleepless nights, at a time when time and energy were scant and precious, we suddenly had to change our diet completely, and restaurants became daunting. I'm pleased to say in the 2 years since I had my second baby, there are so many more options which are readily available, and restaurants have had to up their game, but that doesn't take away from the added anxiety CMPA causes.

Cows' Milk Protein Allergy (CMPA) is an allergy to the cows' milk protein found in all dairy products such as milk, butter, cheese and yoghurt. CMPA is most commonly diagnosed because it leads to the symptoms of baby reflux.

Babies with CMPA need to be assessed by a qualified medical practitioner. If your baby has CMPA then all items with cows' milk protein need to be avoided and in 50% also soya.

Lactose Deficiency is Different to CMPA

CMPA is not the same as lactose intolerance, which is very rare in babies, where there is a lack of 'lactase', the enzyme needed in the gut to break down the naturally occurring lactose sugars which milk contains. Changing to lactose free products is helpful in lactose intolerance, since it removes the lactose, which cannot be digested and causes symptoms. Instead CMPA is an allergy to the actual protein in milk, so changing to lactose free products will not be helpful.

Cow's Milk. Protein. Allergy and Reflux...

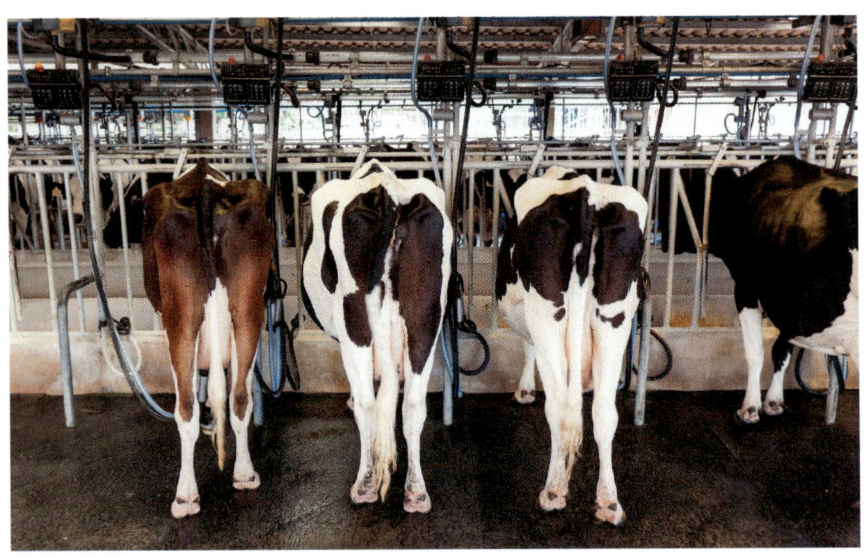

Cow's Milk. Protein. Allergy and Reflux...

Can You Prevent CMPA?

Sadly, as yet, we don't know how to prevent CMPA, but it is fine to consume dairy during your pregnancy. If you have a family history of allergy, hay-fever, asthma, or eczema your baby will have a higher risk of developing CMPA.

When to See a Doctor

It can be really tricky as a new parent to know what is normal with your new baby, and when to see a doctor. Many mums are worried about wasting the doctor's time, but if you have concerns, please don't let this put you off getting your baby checked out.

Book to see your doctor if:

- you have concerns about your baby
- the regurgitation becomes more forceful, and the vomit is expelled with such force that it lands some distance away.
- your baby brings up milk that is green or yellowy green, or if it looks as though it has blood in it.
- your baby has any new problems.
- your baby is very distressed and you can't soothe them.
- your baby can't feed.
- your baby isn't putting on weight.

Cow's Milk. Protein. Allergy and Reflux...

What Will the Doctor Do?

Your doctor will take a history and find out more information about your baby, the vomiting, any additional symptoms and feeding. In some cases, they might arrange for your baby to have some investigations if there is doubt about the diagnosis, or additional concerns.

Can I Change to Goat's Milk Instead?

Goats' milk has proteins which are very similar to the cows' milk protein and so changing to goat milk is very unlikely to help in a baby with CMPA. Approximately 50% of babies with CMPA will also have an allergy to soya as well, since the soya protein is very similar to the cows' milk protein. Therefore, exclusion of soya may well be required.

What Your Doctor Might Prescribe

Previously when a baby was diagnosed with reflux they might have been treated first with anti-reflux medications. A few years ago, this changed and now first line treatment is to exclude an allergic cause. This will mean an exclusion diet for the mother while breastfeeding for at least 4-8 weeks to determine if the symptoms improve.

Cow's Milk Protein Allergy and Reflux...

What Your Doctor Might Prescribe...

In cases where there are still significant symptoms, your doctor might consider a trial of anti-acid medications such as ranitidine or a proton pump inhibitor such as lansoprazole or omeprazole; however, there is limited evidence that these work in children under 1 year of age.

If your baby has been diagnosed with CMPA, have a look at the plant based milk section and what to look out for when you are choosing one.

What is Reflux?

Reflux is the regurgitation of most commonly liquid, back up the oesophagus/food pipe/gullet, from the stomach. There are two types of reflux, 'physiological / functional' and 'non-physiological'. Up to 4 out of 10 babies will have reflux and 9 out of 10 of these will get better by themselves with time.

Physiological Reflux?

Most babies have a degree of physiological reflux, because they spend most of their time lying on their backs. They also have an under-developed muscle ring (sphincter) at the top of their stomach, which fails to prevent regurgitation. This type of reflux is very common, the baby is well, putting on weight appropriately and will naturally improve by their first birthday, as the sphincter muscle develops and the baby becomes more upright.

Postpartum and Beyond

EAT FOR HEALTH

Cow's Milk. Protein. Allergy and Reflux...

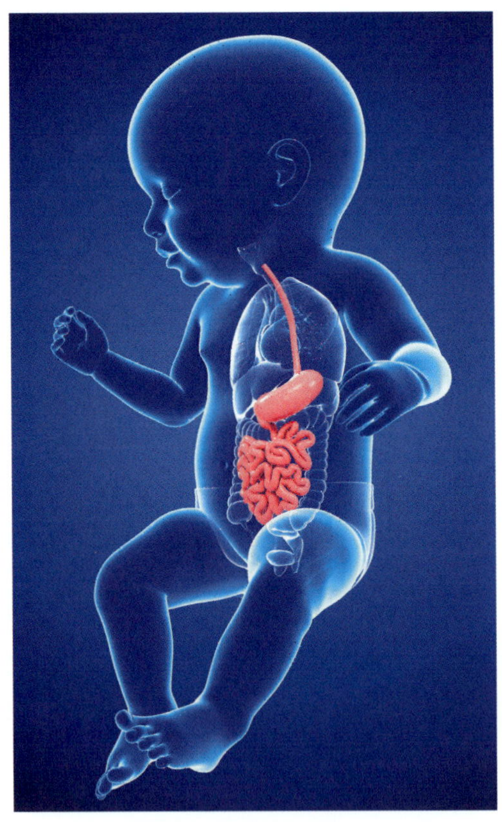

Cow's Milk. Protein. Allergy and Reflux...

Non-physiological Reflux

This refers to reflux which is impacting on the health of the baby and is frequently called Gastro-Oesphageal Reflux Disease (GORD). Recent evidence suggests that allergy, in particular to Cows' Milk Protein, is frequently the cause.

Babies with this type of reflux may have a number of additional symptoms such as:

- being difficult to settle
- arching after feeds and drawing their legs up
- explosive poos or constipation
- blood in their poo
- making rattling noises
- poor weight gain
- coughing or gagging during and after feeds
- frequent vomiting after and between feeds
- eczema before 6 months of age
- cough

Since the regurgitated milk is also mixed with stomach acid, this can create discomfort for the baby. Some babies respond to this discomfort by being put off feeding (termed oral aversion), or want to feed all the time, in an attempt to keep down the acidic milk, and soothe their oesophagus/food pipe.

Most babies will vomit the regurgitated milk, but a minority do not, and this is termed 'silent' reflux. These babies often have milk in their mouth between feeds, from regurgitation even if they don't vomit.

Cow's Milk. Protein. Allergy and Reflux...

Simple Tips To Help Reflux

There are a number of really simple positional changes that can help your baby with the symptoms of reflux:

- elevate the head end of the cot
- avoid placing baby flat even for changing
- hold baby upright after each feed for approximately 20 minutes
- don't bounce your baby, as this is like 'shaking a milk jug', instead soothe by stroking, or swaying
- try a dummy, which helps by drawing the milk down the oesophagus, because of the stimulation of sucking (non-nutritive sucking)
- if you are breastfeeding and have very fast let down or very generous supply, try feeding against gravity by lying on your back, to slow the flow down.

Below is a photo of a mother using a reclining position, lying on her back to breastfeed her baby, because of very fast let down and generous supply.

I found that a wedge, placed under the cot mattress was really helpful to elevate the head of my baby. Remember to abide by the Lullaby Trust Safer Sleep Advice.

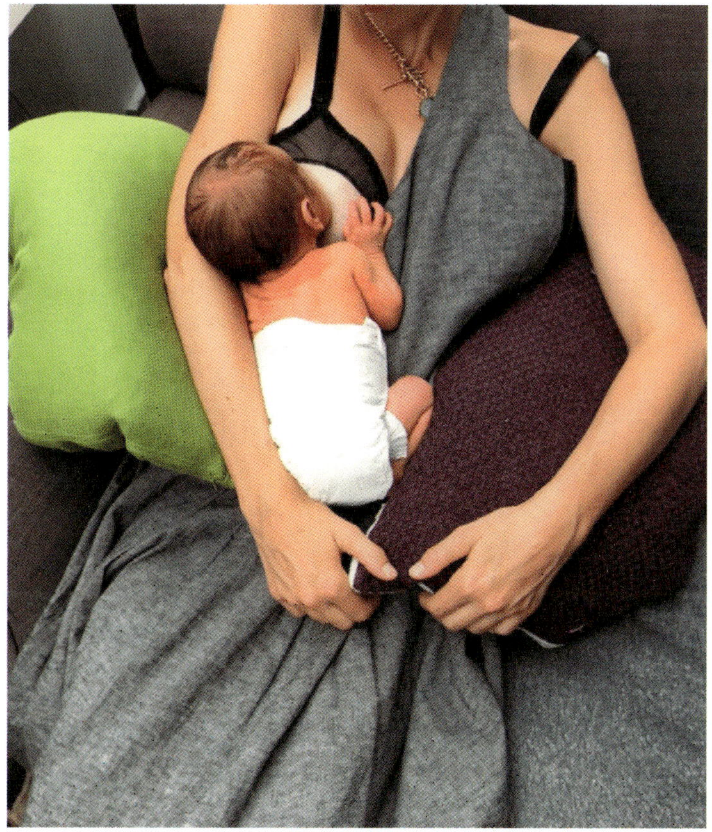

Above is a photo of a mother using a reclining position, lying on her back to breastfeed her baby, because of very fast let down and generous supply.

Cow's Milk. Protein. Allergy and Reflux...

Other Conditions that can be Confused with Reflux

Regurgitation or vomiting can be the final common pathway for a number of other less common medical conditions, ranging from the benign to the more serious including: anatomical problems such as malrotation or hiatus hernia, and infections of both the gastrointestinal system and non-gastrointestinal system.

Over supply of breast milk, while not a medical condition, can also mimic the regurgitation seen in reflux. Additionally, because of the discomfort associated with acid reflux, babies with reflux can be particularly unsettled. Babies with a tongue tie are at risk of 'aerophagia', which means swallowing air as they feed, leading to discomfort from wind, that can mimic the discomfort seen with reflux.

Colic

Colic is used as a catch all term for a baby who is unsettled between 6 weeks to 6 months old and they cry more than 3 hours a day, 3 days a week for at least 1 week. If you are concerned your baby is irritable, or you are unable to soothe them, you should seek medical advice.

Colic and reflux often start at a similar time and can be confused, but a baby with colic has none of the symptoms associated with reflux, and the diagnosis should only be made if your baby is otherwise well.

Cow's Milk. Protein. Allergy and Reflux...

Colic...

There are some simple strategies you can try to soothe your baby with colic:

- swaddle
- rocking
- cuddle them
- winding them
- giving them a warm bath
- white noise
- there is very little evidence to support the use of anti-colic drops or manipulating the bones in your baby's head (cranial osteopathy).

If your baby has been reviewed by a doctor and found to be otherwise well, you might find the purplecrying website useful.

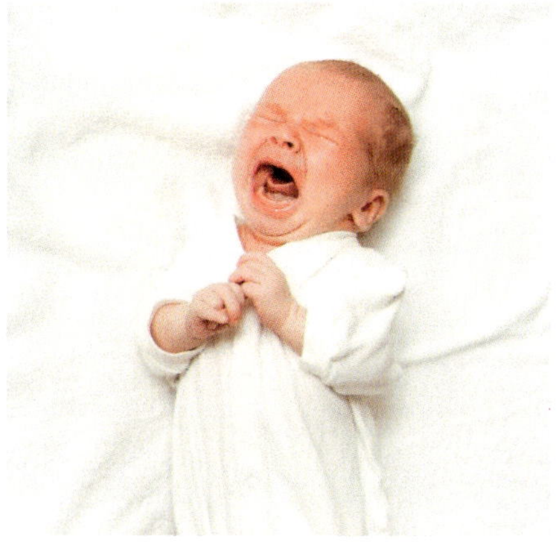

Placental Ingestion - What is the Evidence?

The placenta is a vital organ that enables your baby to grow, providing a supply of nutrients and oxygen. Some women choose to keep their placenta and eat it (placentophagy).

Some have it encapsulated, a process that frequently involves steaming, dehydrating and grinding up the placenta, before turning it into capsules. While others eat it raw, cooked, or dehydrated, by itself or added to smoothies or food.

Some people believe that there are benefits to ingesting the placenta including:

- increased breastmilk production
- restoration of iron levels post birth
- decrease in postnatal depression
- increase in the hormone oxytocin, which helps the uterus contract back down to a non-pregnant size. Oxytocin is commonly called the love hormone, and is involved in bonding.
- Ingestion of corticotrophin-releasing hormone (CRH), a hormone involved in the stress response.

The precise role of placental CRH is unknown, but it does appear to be involved in gestational length, acting as a clock, and communication between the foetus and mother.

Levels of CRH are also frequently elevated in pathological conditions of pregnancy where foetal wellbeing is compromised. CRH is involved in the corticosteroid feedback loop, so that when steroids are produced, this stimulates production of CRH by the placenta, which then feedback to glucocorticoid receptors in the pituitary gland (in the brain), to reduce the stimulation to produce more steroid hormones.

Placental Ingestion - What is the Evidence?

Even though placental ingestion has been performed in some cultures for hundreds of years, there is very little scientific evidence. A randomised controlled trial compare placental encapsulation versus placebo, and found that no difference in maternal mood, bonding or fatigue were observed. Convincing data or even placebo controlled randomised trials are lacking.

Cooked or steamed placenta will likely denature (permanently unravel and destroy the function of) the hormones, so that ingestion is unlikely to have an effect. Also the presumed nutrients' contained in the placenta are not present in sufficiently high concentrations to be potentially beneficial to the mother postpartum.

While the reports of benefits, come from self-reported claims, there are a number of possible risks associated with placental ingestion:

- infection
- accumulation of environmental toxins
- increased risk of blood clot from estrogen in the placental tissue
- contamination during handling / processing

The placenta is like any other organ and will start to degrade as soon as it is removed from the body. It must be refrigerated and stored carefully like other raw meat product to prevent pathogenic infection. Like any blood product, blood borne diseases can be passed on by incorrect handling of the placenta and this needs to be considered if friends or family members also ingest it.

There is no regulation of commercial placental encapsulation or preparation services, so if you decide to consider using such a service, ensure that high food hygiene standards are met.

Placental Ingestion - What is the Evidence?

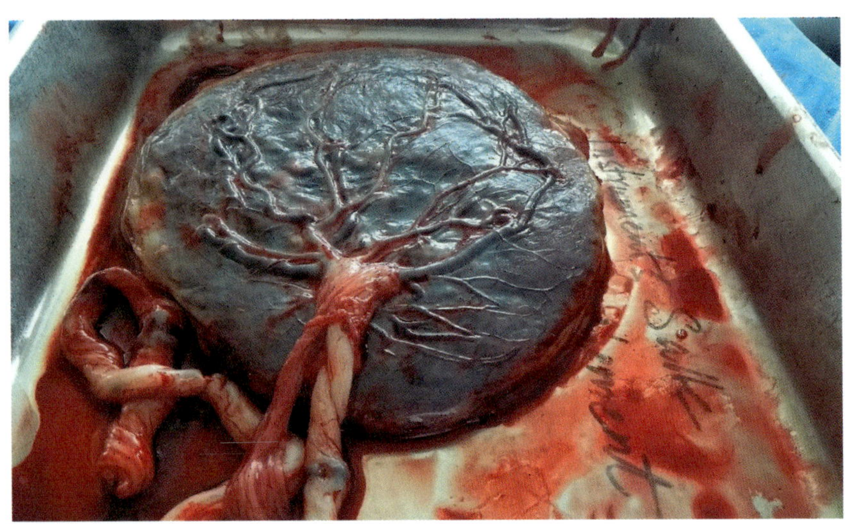

Tips for Helping with Constipation

Constipation is common during pregnancy for a number of reasons. Firstly progesterone, a key hormone in pregnancy has the effect of slowing the natural movement of the gut, which makes constipation more likely.

Secondly, many women find that they will be affected by feeling sick in the first trimester and so less likely to eat the 30g of fibre a day that they need.

Thirdly, as your baby grows inside of you, everything else is a bit squashed, slowing the passage of food in your gut. Finally, it is easy to become dehydrated in pregnancy, because you need more fluid than usual, as your blood supply increases.

Once you have had your baby, constipation can still be a common problem with many women understandably fearing 'the first poo', especially if you have a tear or surgical wound.

If you were already a bit constipated during pregnancy, try to prioritise eating fibre and keeping hydrated, so that the first poo post birth isn't so daunting. If you are in pain, then my advice would be to take adequate pain relief (paracetamol and ibuprofen are safe during breastfeeding) so that you don't put off going to the toilet, as this can make it even worse when you do try.

Eat more:

- fruit and vegetables
- bran
- wholegrain carbohydrates
- legumes
- pulses
- drink plenty of water (approximately 8 x 200ml glasses per day.

Should I Choose Organic Food?

I'm commonly asked this question about organic food, with the assumption being that organic food must be safer. While non organic food is produced with herbicides and pesticides, these are within limits that are safe for consumption.

The nutritional differences between organic and non-organic food is minimal, but widespread use of antibiotics and herbicide chemicals may have effects, even though they are within safe limits.

While there currently is not sufficient enough evidence to support a strong statement on the benefits of organic food, there is a growing evidence of health benefits.

A recent meta-analysis where multiple trials were combined and analysed together, found that an increased organic intake was associated with reduced incidence of infertility, birth defects, allergies, ear infections, pre-eclampsia, metabolic syndrome, high BMI, and non-Hodgkin lymphoma.

One of the problems with studies looking at possible health benefits of organic food, is that people that choose to eat organic food, are more likely to make healthier lifestyle choices in general.

This makes it difficult to interpret whether health benefits are related to lifestyle changes other than organic food.

Tips

- organic food may be associated with health benefits
- other healthier lifestyle choices maybe be just as, if not more important
- organic food is unlikely to pose any risk, except the cost implications.

Which Vitamins Does Your Baby Need?

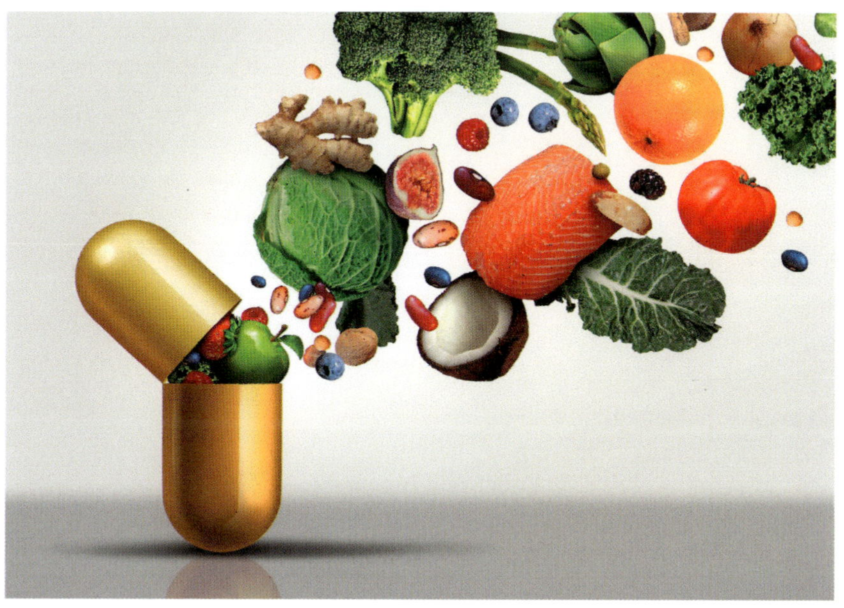

Which Vitamins Does Your Baby Need?

This depends on a number of different factors, including their age, and how much formula milk they drink per day. Vitamins for children can be a confusing topic. Who needs what, when do you start, how long do you carry on for? I'll talk you through the guidance as there are different groups needing different support.

Vitamin D

Vitamin D though found in limited amounts in oily fish and eggs, is primarily manufactured in our bodies by exposure to sunlight. Therefore, as it is important to keep your baby or child safe out of the sun, most children will need a supplement. I like the Better you vitamin spray for infants suitable from birth to 3 years old.

Babies

All breastfeeding babies should be started on a supplement of Vitamin D from birth, regardless of whether mum is taking a supplement or not. The recommended dose is 8.5-10 micrograms (mcg) per day. Babies who are having more than 500mls of formula per day, do not need any vitamin supplements, because the formula is fortified with supplementary vitamins including vitamin D.

Children

Once your baby is over 12 months, they should take a vitamin D supplement of 10 micrograms (mcg) per day until they are 4 years old (unless your child still has more than 500mls of formula a day).

Which Vitamins Does Your Baby Need?

Vitamin A

Vitamin A is important for night time vision, the immune system and skin health.
Foods rich in vitamin A are:

- dark green vegetables such as spinach, cabbage and broccoli
- dairy products
- carrots, sweet potatoes, swede
- liver
- some oils
- fortified spreads

From 6 months to 5 years old, it is recommended that children take a supplement of vitamin A, unless they are taking more than 500mls of formula per day.

Vitamin C

Vitamin C is important for immune system, and general health. The absorption of iron can be increased by combining foods rich in vitamin C at the same meal.

Foods rich in vitamin C are:

- berries
- oranges
- kiwi fruit
- bell peppers
- broccoli

From 6 months to 5 years old, it is recommended that children take supplement of vitamin C, unless they are taking more than 500mls of formula per day.

Which Vitamins Does Your Baby Need?

Vitamin B

The B vitamin complex consists of a number of different compounds. For children weaned onto a vegan diet, they need to supplement B12. Otherwise, there are no recommendations for children to take B vitamin supplements, as they should meet their requirements through their diet alone. However, B vitamins are often included in multivitamins.

Omega 3

Omega 3 is a type of fat, that has to be consumed in our diet, and cannot be manufactured in our bodies. It is found it oily fish such as salmon, cod, mackerel, trout, haddock, plaice and pollack and also nuts, vegetable oils, seeds, and tofu.

Current recommendations are to include one to two portions of oily fish in your own and children's diet every week.

The following is a guide to approximate portion sizes of oily fish:

- 18m to 3 years = 1 -3 tablespoons or 1/4 - 3/4 small fillet
- 4 - 6 years = 2-4 tablespoons or 1/2 - 1 small fillet
- 7 - 11 years = 3 - 5 tablespoons or 1 -1 1/2 small fillets
- 12 years to adult = 140g fresh fish or 1 small can of oily fish

There are currently no recommendations for adults or children to take omega 3 supplements, but there has been evidence of some benefit in specific groups of adults.

Which Vitamins Does Your Baby Need?

Omega 3...

If you decide to supplement your child's diet with Omega 3 supplements you should consider the following:

- choose an Omega-3 supplement rather than a fish liver oil.
- choose an age appropriate supplement for your child
- omega 3 supplements frequently contain vitamin A. The Scientific Advisory Committee on Nutrition (SACN) advises that if you take supplements containing vitamin A such as fish liver oils, you should not have more than a total of 1.5mg (1500ug) a day from food and supplements combined.
- seek advice if you are unsure.

Iron

Most toddlers do not need to take iron supplements, however there are some groups that are higher risk, and more likely to need to supplement their diet; these are babies with low (<2.5Kg) and very low birth weight.

All children should be offered an iron-rich diet (meat and iron-fortified foods) from 6m and drink less than 500mls of cows milk per day. This is because if your toddler fills up on milk, they will eat less solid food, and miss out on foods containing iron. If you are concerned, then seek medical advice.

Which Vitamins Does Your Baby Need?

Summary

If your child or baby has 500mls of formula per day, they do not need any vitamin supplements.

Breast fed babies should take vitamin D supplements from birth to aged 4 years. At 6 months they should also be started on vitamin A and C supplements until aged 4 years.

I like the Better You multivitamin sprays for infants, suitable from 1 to 3 years.

Aim for up to 1-2 portions of oily fish per week to meet omega 3 needs.

There is no need to supplement other vitamins, as their needs should be met by their diet, unless your child excludes food groups such a dairy free or vegan diets.

Postpartum and Beyond

EAT FOR HEALTH

A Practical Guide to Starting Weaning

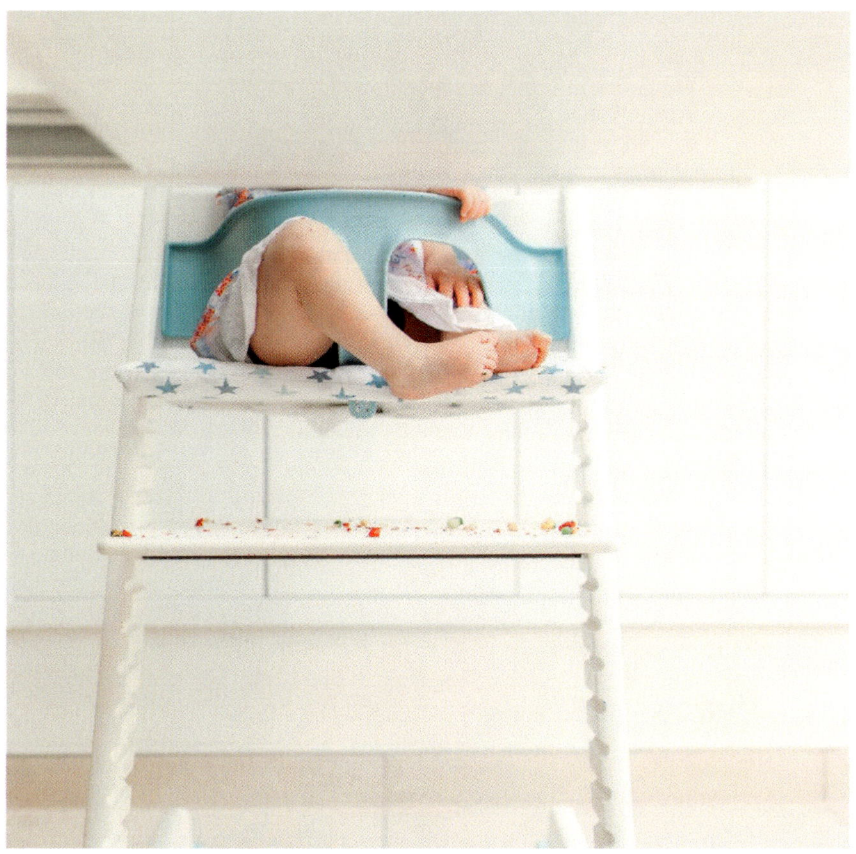

A Practical Guide to Starting Weaning

Introducing food to your baby can be an exciting but daunting time for many parents and you may have many questions.

When is My Baby Ready for Weaning?

Government advice in the UK is to start weaning from around 6 months (but not before 4 months of age). However, in reality when a baby is ready to start weaning, will vary, as they will all reach their developmental milestones at a slightly different pace.

It's a good idea to wait until they are ready, because they are more likely to be able to move food safely around their mouth. For the first 6 months, milk (breast or formula) provides all their nutrition. After this time while milk still provides most of their nutrients, they do start to need additional intake of some micronutrients, such as iron. This why weaning is sometimes called complementary feeding, as it complements the nutrients from milk.

These are the signs to look out for that your baby is ready to start trying food:

- can stay in a sitting position and hold their head steady
- can coordinate their eyes, hands and mouth so that they can look at their food, pick it up and put it in their mouth
- can swallow food, instead of just spitting it back out

Some behaviours can be mistaken for signs of being ready for food, these are:

- chewing their fists
- wanting extra milk feeds, as they might just be going through a growth spurt waking up in the night more than usual.

A Practical Guide to Starting Weaning

When is My Baby Ready for Weaning?...

Sadly starting food is not more likely to help your baby sleep through the night. Have a look for the three main signs and that they are happening regularly, not just a one off.

My Baby was Premature

Babies who were born prematurely, should in general follow the same guidance, and still start when they are ready, around 6 months corrected. This means 6 months from the time they were due to be born. For additional guidance you should speak with your GP or health visitor.

What Time of Day Should I Start?

While there is no set time that you should start introducing foods to your baby, you will probably find them more receptive if they are not tired or hungry. So to start with offer your baby milk first, and then as they get used to eating, you can change this to before milk.

Morning can be a great time too, as if your baby has any new symptoms such as an allergic reaction, it can be less scary and more visible than in the evening at bed time.

Playing and exploring food is completely normal for babies, so expect lots of mess, and leave plenty of time. Babies copy other people's behaviour, so it is also a good idea to sit down at the same time and eat with your baby, modelling the behaviour you would like them to learn.

Postpartum and Beyond

EAT FOR HEALTH

A Practical Guide to Starting Weaning

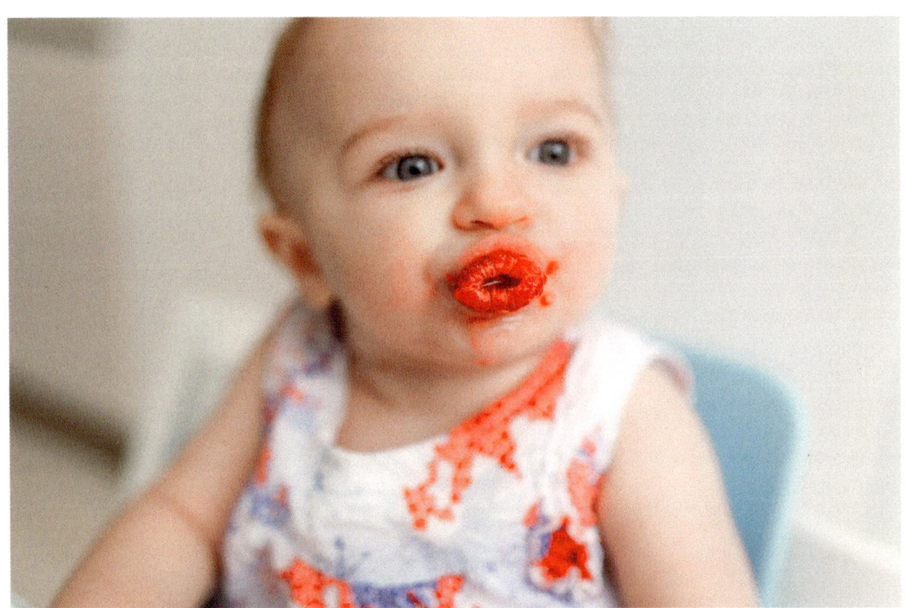

A Practical Guide to Starting Weaning

Do I Need Any Equipment?

Before you start weaning, there are a few things that you need to get, but you really don't need a fancy steamer or blender to weaning your baby. A potato masher is a cheaper way to make purees if you don't have a blender. BLW requires even less equipment, only some of the food will require adaptation for your baby.

There is really only one essential item and that is a high chair, preferably one where your baby can be supported to sit upright, safely strapped in, ideally with their feet flat on a support. My favourite is the Stoke Trip Trap chair, as it provides all these features, and grows with your baby and child, providing an ergonomic position for time at the kitchen table.

Once you start offering complementary food, also do the same with water using a free flowing sippy cup. Soft spoons are better for baby's gums than metal spoons, and can be used for purées.

I'd recommend using a bowl that bounces, as you will probably find it on the floor at some point, or one with suction. I also love the silicon plate that has suction to the table, but also has a lid. This makes it easy to prepare food and take it out with you.

Try to get a bib that is easy to clean. I found one with sleeves the best as weaning can be very messy!

A Practical Guide to Starting Weaning

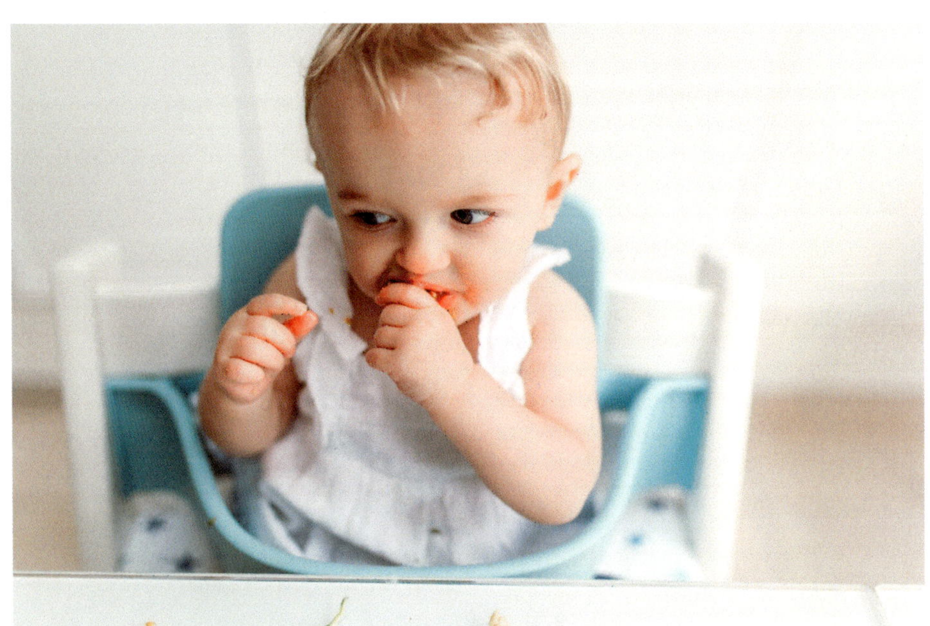

A Practical Guide to Starting Weaning

Baby Led or Purée or Both?

There is no evidence that your baby is more likely to choke doing baby led weaning. However, doing a baby first aid course can be useful and reassuring before you start weaning. Also St John's Ambulance have a useful video on choking (https://www.sja.org.uk/get-advice/first-aid-advice/choking/baby-choking/).

Baby lead weaning (BLW) means using mostly finger foods that your baby can explore and try at their own speed. While some of the foods will need additional preparation to make them safer, there is no need to purée the food.

Whether you choose to try BWL or purées or use a mixture of both is up to you. Many parents find that BLW can be easier, as your baby can share most of your food, meaning less preparation. In addition, babies are more in control of regulating their own food intake with appetite, and therefore have a decreased risk of obesity later in life.

There are less likely to be meal time battles, and be associated with less fussy eating. However, there are risks with BLW, such that babies may eat less than being spoon fed, and therefore risk not eating enough iron rich food. You can avoid this by aiming to offer an easy to eat, iron rich source of food at each meal time.

A Practical Guide to Starting Weaning

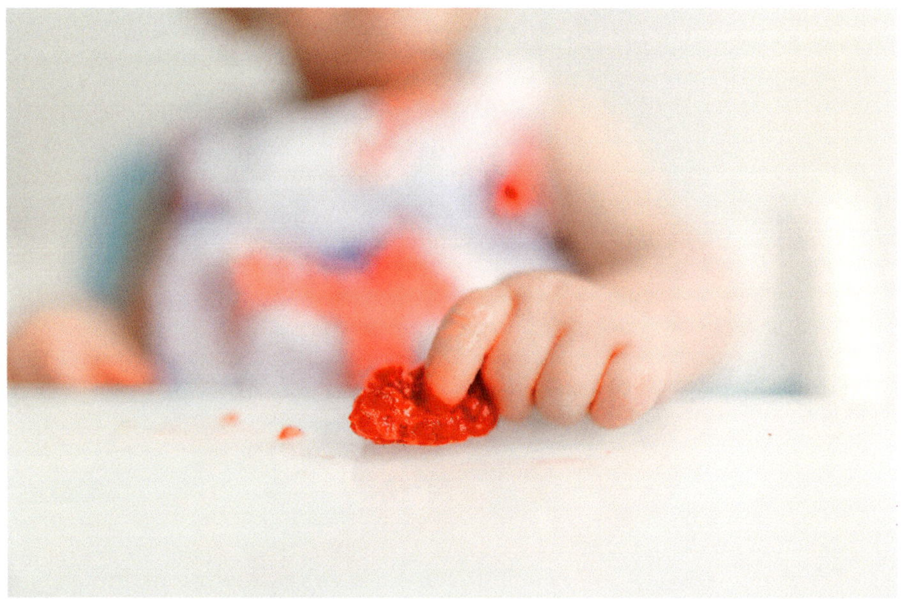

A Practical Guide to Starting Weaning

How to Prepare Food for BLW

You might feel a bit lost at the thought of just handing your baby a piece of broccoli, but there are a few ways of preparing food to decrease the risk of choking:

- food should be about the size of an adult finger and not easy to break off (such as a raw apple or carrot – instead, try coarsely grating these)
- round or cylindrical foods such as grapes and sausages should be cut longitudinally into halves or quarters to begin with. Round berries like blueberries can be squashed with your fingers or a fork to reduce the choking risk. Sausages should have the skin removed and cut longitudinally (not into disks).
- for harder vegetables and pasta, cook these until they are nice and soft.
- babies when they start weaning, will not have a pincer grip where they can pick up something small like a pea, instead they need to be able to grip the item in the palm of their hand. Strips of food are easier to hold this way, and for slippery foods such as bananas and avocados, leaving some skin on as a handle can help them grip it.

Purées and Textures

If you chose to offer your baby purees then the guidance is to start with smooth purées and move onto progressively lumpier food as they grow

- 6 months (not before 4 months): smooth purées
- 7-9 months: mashed food with some lumps
- 9-12 months: mashed, minced and chopped family meals

A Practical Guide to Starting Weaning

Which Foods Should I Offer First?

Vegetables are a great way to start weaning, especially those that are not naturally sweet such as broccoli florets, spinach, cooked courgette sticks, cooked carrot sticks, cauliflower florets and avocados (technically a fruit not a vegetable).

Starting with fruit, risks your baby being less keen on trying foods that aren't as naturally sweet like vegetables, that they will need to learn to like. Harder vegetables may need to be cooked a bit more, so that they are nice and soft for your baby to gum.

Once your baby has started on vegetables, add in a range of different fruits and foods which are higher risk for allergies (see below). As you establish a routine, regardless of how you are offering food, (whether that is finger food or purées), think about offering items from different vegetables, fruit, carbohydrates, and protein (and iron).

Carbohydrate finger food ideas:

- oat biscuit
- plain cracker
- pitta bread strip
- bread/toast finger
- cooked pasta shapes
- strips of pancakes (without added sugar, such as banana or sweet potato pancakes)

A Practical Guide to Starting Weaning

Which Foods Should I Offer First...

Protein (and iron) finger food ideas:

- strips of omelette or lumps of scrambled egg
- cooked chicken or turkey pieces
- crushed beans (broad beans, chickpeas, kidney beans) – crushing reduces risk of choking
- flakes or pieces of white fish
- pieces of cheese
- cooked beef pieces
- strips of tofu

Allergenic Foods

Some foods are higher risk than others for causing an allergic reaction. These are:

- eggs
- wheat
- fish and seafood
- seeds
- cow's milk
- tree nuts
- peanuts (these are actually legumes like soya and lentils and are different to tree nuts!)

Once you baby is happily eating vegetables and fruit, you can start to add in these allergenic foods, in small quantities, one at a time. This is because if there is a reaction, the trigger food can be easily identified. There is now evidence that introducing these allergenic foods earlier is of benefit.

A Practical Guide to Starting Weaning

Foods to Avoid

Try to avoid your baby foods that have added sugar or salt so avoid chocolate, sweets, sugary drinks, salt in stock cubes, cakes, biscuits, breakfast cereals with honey or added sugar.

Honey should also be avoided in babies less than a year of age, as there is a risk of botulism from spores naturally present in honey.

Is My Baby a Fussy Eater?

Your baby might turn their nose up at new foods when you introduce them, but this does not mean that they are a fussy eater. Instead babies need to be introduced to foods multiple times before they accept them.

This is true for toddlers too when they are still learning new foods. Keep introducing new items along side others that you know they like.

Postpartum and Beyond

EAT FOR HEALTH

Top Tips for Weaning

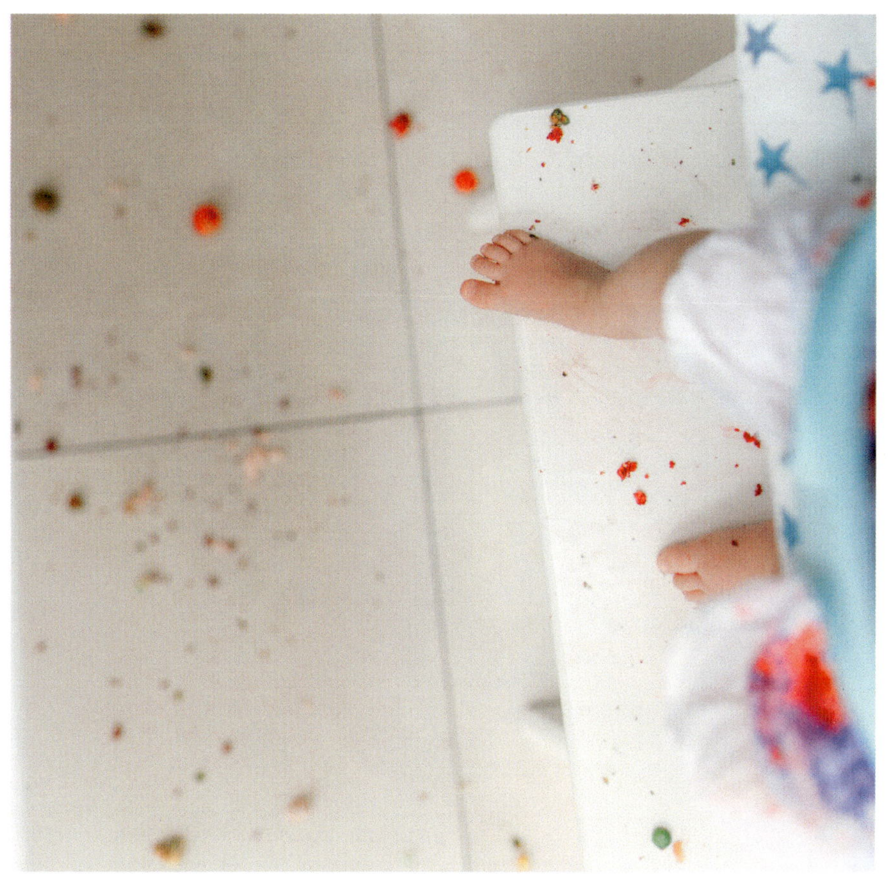

Top Tips for Weaning

Its ok to feel a bit nervous about starting weaning, with lots of information to take on board, and potential worries about food allergies or choking. These are my top tips for making the weaning process as fun and enjoyable as possible:

- keep calm, as your baby is an expert at picking up your stress. The happier and more relaxed you are, the more likely your baby will be the same. If you feel stressed, try turning on some calming music to help you feel more relaxed.

- eat with friends and family: eating with and watching other people eat is a great way to model positive behaviour to your child. It's one of the reasons many children eat different food at nursery, that they might refuse at home! Food isn't just about the nutrients, it's also about establishing a positive routine, and importance of the social benefits of sitting together for a meal.

- make it fun: try going on a picnic or making a face with the food. Even for adults, how food is presented, is important. Offer a variety of food of different tastes, textures, and colours to keep the weaning journey exciting.

- avoid distractions: try to focus on offering and enjoying food together. It is better if your child can learn to enjoy food, and listen to their body so that they stop when they are full. This is less likely if there are distractions like toys or TV.

- let them explore: try to avoid stopping your baby exploring their food and accept that weaning is messy. Children learn through smell, touch, and looking at food. This is important for them to establish acceptance of food.

Top Tips for Weaning...

- establish a routine: most children respond well to routines, so that they can predict what will happen next. As you become more familiar with weaning, and find a routine, your baby will be able to predict when to expect food.

- always stay with your child while they are eating, ensure they are sitting up right, with their feet supported, and you chop up foods that are a particular choking hazard like tomatoes and grapes.

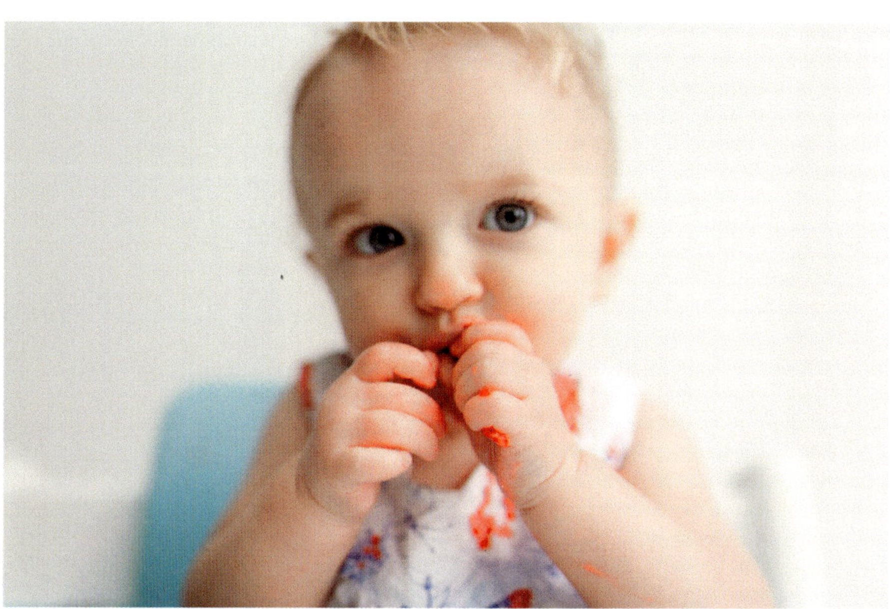

Vegan and Vegetarian Weaning

Vegan diets are increasingly popular in adults with now up to 10% of adults reported as vegan, increasingly children are being weaned onto a vegan diet. You might be considering this yourself for your baby, and be worried about possible risks, or put off from well-meaning friends and family telling you they need meat and dairy.

Vegan diets are high in fibre and low in fat. While a high fibre diet in adults is beneficial, for children, it can mean that they fill up quickly before they get the calories they need. Children also need a higher fat diet than adults. All people following a vegan diet are also at risk of being deficient for vitamin B12, and iron. Having said this, it is perfectly safe to raise your child on a vegan diet, it just requires a bit more thought and planning to ensure that you adequately meet their nutritional needs. If you plan to wean your baby onto a vegan diet, when they are little it can be difficult to get enough vitamin B12, riboflavin, iron, zinc, calcium and iron so they might need to take supplements so speak to your GP.

If you are concerned your child is filling up on high fibre food and not getting enough calories and nutrients, try these tips:

- offer more high calorie foods such as hummus, nut butters, seed butters, tahini, full fat yoghurts
- mix unsaturated oils such as extra virgin olive oil or avocado oil into food and drizzle more on the top before serving
- add extra tahini and extra virgin olive oil to hummus.

Postpartum and Beyond

EAT FOR HEALTH

Vegan and Vegetarian Weaning

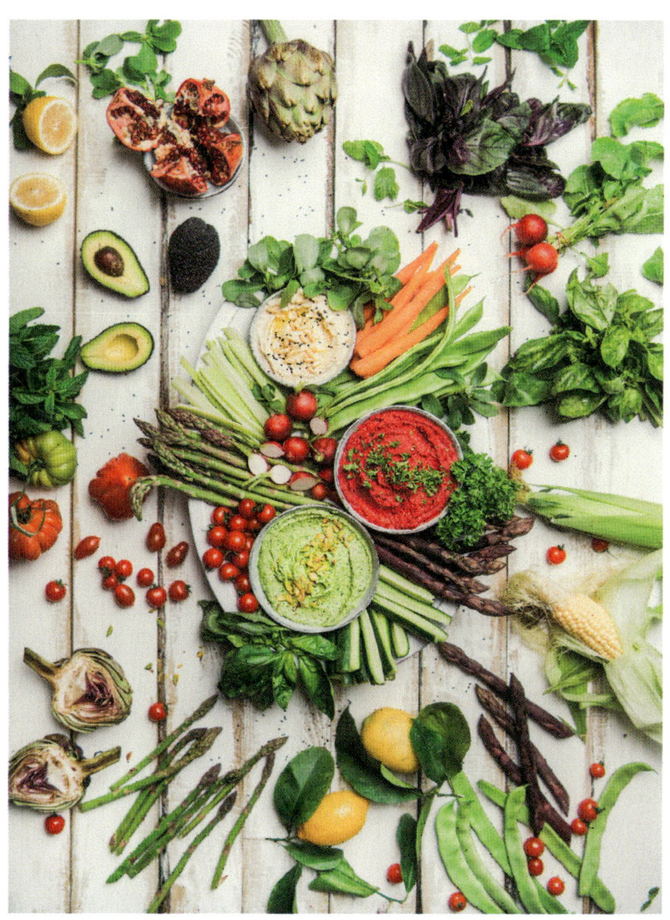

Vegan and Vegetarian Weaning

Vitamin B12

Vitamin B12 is usually found in animal products such as dairy, eggs and meat. Children on a vegan or vegetarian diet will need to take supplementary B12, or eat enough foods that are fortified with vitamin B12, such as breakfast cereals, some alternative diary free yoghurt and milk. alternatives.

Yeast extracts also contain B12, but try to avoid brands containing salt for younger children. Nutritional yeast also contains B12, and can be great sprinkled on top of food or mixed in to create a cheesy taste.

Iodine

Iodine is mainly found in dairy and fish, but is found in much smaller quantities in cereals and grains. Levels vary considerably due to how much iodine is found in the soil where the plants are grown. Some plant based milks have just started to fortify their products with iodine, which is a great way to get enough iodine.

Seaweed and some kelp products contain very high levels of iodine and are not recommended. If you or your baby are unable to get enough iodine through your diet, you might need to consider a supplement.

Vegan and Vegetarian Weaning

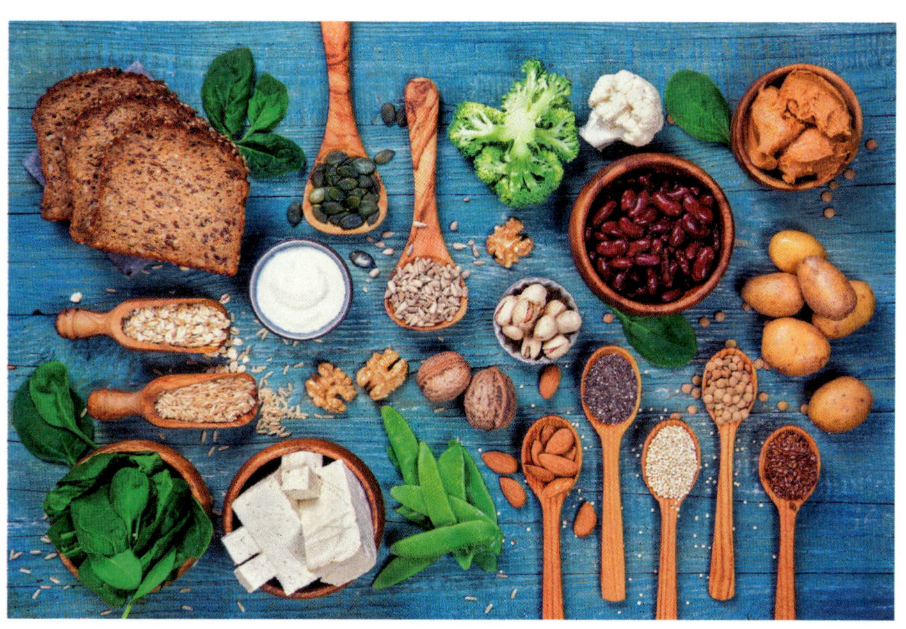

Vegan and Vegetarian Weaning

Iron

Iron is needed to make red blood cells to carry the oxygen around your body. If you are deficient, this can lead to symptoms of tiredness and ultimately poor growth.
Iron rich vegan foods are:

- pulses and legumes such as beans, lentils, and chickpeas
- dark green vegetables
- nuts and seeds - (avoid whole nuts in children under 5 years old to reduce the risk of choking, and try nut butters or ground instead)
- wholegrains like brown rice and wholemeal bread
- dried fruit such as prunes, figs, apricots
- fortified breakfast cereals

The absorption of non-haem (plant based) iron is enhanced by vitamin C. Iron deficiency is common in both vegan and vegetarian diets, so this food combination may be helpful.

Omega 3

Omega 3 fatty acids are essential for health and cannot be produced in the body, so must be included in your diet. They are commonly found in oily fish, but plant based sources are:

- seeds such as flaxseed, chia and hemp seeds
- walnuts - (avoid whole nuts in children under 5 years old to reduce the risk of choking, and try ground instead)
- for vegetarian children eggs that are enriched with omega 3

There is evidence that suggests that plant based sources of omega 3 fatty acids may not have the same health benefits for reducing the risk of heart disease as those found in oily fish.

Vegan and Vegetarian Weaning

Calcium

While dairy products are a good source of calcium, non-organic plant based milk alternatives are now frequently fortified with calcium (see the plant based milk section).

From the start of weaning, cow's milk can be used for cooking. From 1 year of age, children can be offered cow's milk or an unsweetened plant based milk alternative that is fortified with calcium. Rice milks should be avoided in all children under the age of 5 years old because they contain too much arsenic.

Other plant based sources of calcium are:

- tahini – sesame paste
- almond butter
- tofu set with calcium
- fortified bread
- pulses such as beans, chickpeas and lentils
- dried figs
- green leafy vegetables such as cabbage, kale and broccoli.

Protein

All proteins are made up of smaller building block called amino acids. There are 22 different amino acids. Of these 13 can be synthesised within our bodies, while 9 can not, and have to be eaten. These are called essential amino acids, as we need them to survive. Meat and fish contain all the essential amino acids and are therefore called 'complete' protein sources.

Vegan and Vegetarian Weaning

Protein...

Most vegetables are not complete protein sources, except for example chia seeds, buckwheat, soya, hemp and quinoa.

This means that people eating a vegetarian or vegan diet must combine protein sources in order to get adequate amounts of all the essential amino acids during each day. The non-essential amino acids can be synthesised by your body in the liver from nitrogen, fats and carbohydrates.

Eating a diet with a wide variety of protein sources will help you to get adequate amounts of all the essential acids each day.

Good plant based protein sources are:

- hummus
- tofu
- beans
- chickpeas
- lentils
- soya product
- nuts and seeds - (avoid whole nuts in children under 5 years old to reduce the risk of choking, and try ground instead).

Vegan and Vegetarian Weaning

Carbohydrates

While wholegrain carbohydrates are better for health, and you are usually advised to avoid refined carbohydrates such as white bread and pasta, children under the age of 5 years old are advised not to only eat wholegrains. This is because they can fill up on high fibre foods such as wholegrains before they have had enough calories and nutrients. This is especially important for children on a vegetarian or vegan diet.

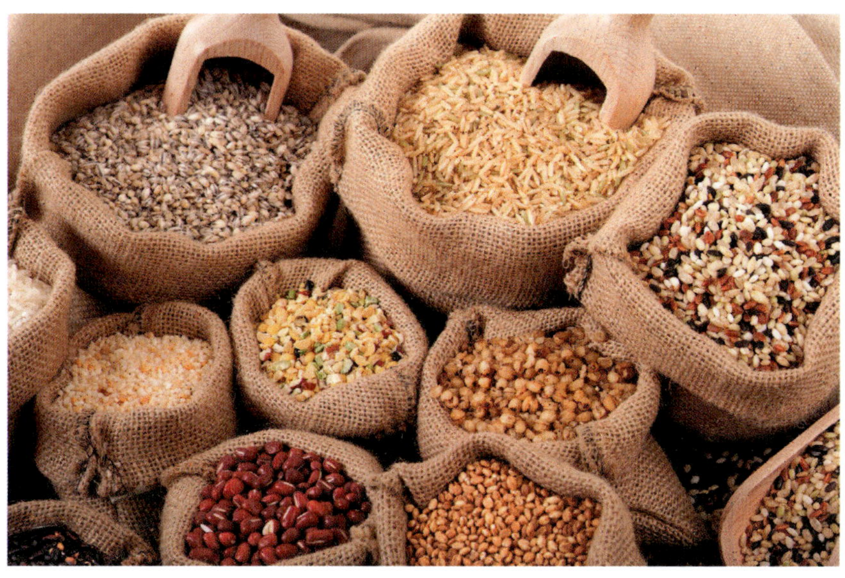

How to Divide Up Your Child's Plate

As a general rule when feeding your child (aged between 1-4 years), it can be easier to think of the day as a whole and how many portions of each food groups you should offer. Depending on whether your child eats more at meals, or needs more snacks, then you can divide them up according to your child's needs.

During the day, aim to offer the following:

- 5 portions of starchy foods
- 5 portions of fruit and vegetables (fresh, frozen, dried and canned all count)
- 3 portions of dairy
- 2 portions of protein (3 if your child is vegetarian or vegan)

Over the week, aim to offer 2 portions of fish, including one oily fish such as salmon or mackerel.

Offer approximately 6-8 cups (150-200mls per cup) of milk or water at meal and snack times.

Try to avoid fizzy drinks or neat fruit juice and instead dilute fruit juice to 1 part juice and 10 parts water.

Salty foods such as olives and baked beans should be limited so that your child has less than 2g of salt per day. If possible try to avoid food with added salt such as crisps, or processed meat and use herbs for flavour instead of salt.

How to Choose a Plant Based Milk

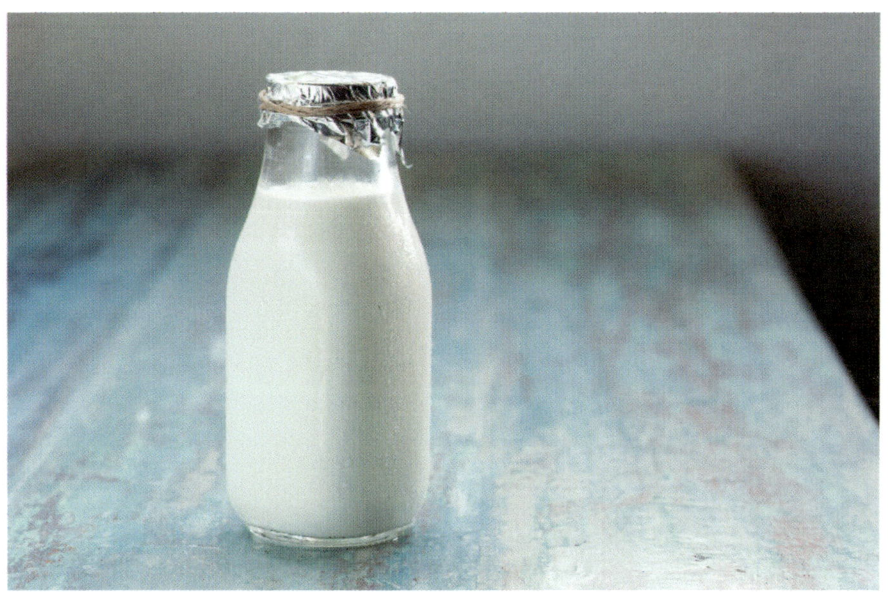

How to Choose a Plant Based Milk

I'm often asked by clients about dairy free or plant based milks. Five years ago I gave up dairy and soya products while breastfeeding my son who had cows milk protein allergy (CMPA).

Now there are far more milks to choose from, and they are much more easily available. Most high street coffee shops and cafes will now have at least one dairy free version available. Lots of options though, means lots of choice. So how do you choose a plant based milk?

- There are lots of different types of 'milk', primarily made from nuts, coconut, oats, soya.
- They all taste pretty different, so shop around until you find a milk you like.
- Try and avoid those with carrageenan as there is some evidence this is a stomach irritant.
- Hazelnut milk is delicious for making hot chocolate, but isn't fortified with calcium.
- Choose one that is unsweetened.
- Oatly Whole and barista foam really well, and are great for making coffee. They also don't split and curdle in tea.
- Infants that have CMPA can be changed onto a plant based milk such as Oatly whole (which is fortified and high in fat) from 12 months provided they are growing well.
- 50% of babies with CMPA are also allergic to soya, as the protein structure is very similar.
- When you chose a milk for children over 12 months, look for an unsweetened milk, that is high in calories, fat and protein, and is fortified with calcium and iodine.

Keep reading to see which I recommend and why.

How to Choose a Plant Based Milk

Iodine

Until recently iodine has been largely thought to be sufficient in our diets. However, research has raised concerns that pregnant and breastfeeding women are at risk of deficiency. Dairy products and fish are iodine rich foods, so people following a vegan diet are at risk of iodine deficiency.

Depending on your life stage, people need different amounts of iodine per day:

- Children 1-8years need 90 µg
- Children 9-13 years need 120 µg
- Teenagers 14-18 years and adults need 150µg
- Pregnant and breastfeeding women need 200 µg

See my comparison table below to see which milks contain iodine and how much.

Calcium

Calcium in our diets is incredibly important for our bone, teeth and muscle health. For many people most of their calcium requirement comes from eating dairy products. Therefore, it can be difficult to get enough calcium with dairy exclusion. If you are following a dairy-free diet, I recommend looking for a plant based milk that is fortified with calcium for your main milk.

How to Choose a Plant Based Milk

Calcium...

Depending on your life stage, people need different amounts of calcium per day:

- children 1-3 years 350mg
- children 4-6 years 450mg
- children 7-10 years 550mg
- female adolescents 11-18 years 800mg
- male adolescents 11-18 years 1000mg
- adults 19 + years 700mg
- breastfeeding mothers 1250mg
- pre menopausal women 700mg
- post menopausal women 1200mg
- women with Coeliac disease or Inflammatory bowel disease 1000-1500mg.

See the Calcium section and the nutrition planner at the end of this book for practical advice on calcium rich foods and drinks.

Nutrients in Milk

While micronutrients are important in milk alternatives, so are macronutrients (carbohydrates, fat and protein). For children milk is an important nutrient source, and so consideration of the levels of macronutrients in the milk is important.

As an adult you might decide to look for a lower fat and calorie alternative, it is different for children.

How to Choose a Plant Based Milk

Nutrients in Milk...

Over the age of 12 months, when cow's milk and plant based alternatives can be introduced, it is generally recommended that you look for one that resembles cow's milk as closely as possible in terms of macronutrients. I've combined a handy table below of the majority of milks on the market and compared their energy (Kilo Calories), protein, fat, calcium and iodine content.

I've ranked these in order of preference based on their overall macronutrient and micronutrient content. You can see that full fat cow's milk has the highest levels of macronutrients when energy, fat, and protein content are taken together compared with the other milk alternatives. However, other milks do have higher calcium levels and added iodine.

Here is a handy list of the commonly available milks in the United Kingdom and their macro and micronutrient content per 100mls of milk (approximately a 1/3 of a cup).

How to Choose a Plant Based Milk

Nutrients in Milk

Per 100ml of milk	Calcium (mg)	Iodine (µg)	Fat (g)	Calories Kcal	Protein (g)
Plenish organic unsweetened soya	145	30	2.9	47	3.7
Oatly Whole	120	22.5	2.8	57	1
Marks and Spencer's unsweetened soya	120	30	2	39	3.4
Alpro Fresh Original Soya Milk Alternative	120	22.5	1.8	39	3
Plenish organic unsweetened almond	153	30.08	3	32	1
Marks and Spencer's oat	120	30	1.6	49	0.5
Plenish organic unsweetened oat	145	30	1	41	0.4
Marks and Spencer's sweetened almond	120	30	1.1	39	0.5
Marks and Spencer's coconut	120	30	1.9	29	0.2
Marks and Spencer's unsweetened almond	120	30	1.1	17	0.4
Full fat cows milk	124	0	4	69	3.5
The Mighty Society unsweetened pea mylk	186	0	2	35	3.2
KoKo dairy free unsweetened chilled	120	0	1.3	15	0.7
Rebel Kitchen whole	0	0	5.5	75	0.8
Rude Health Ultimate Organic Almond	0	0	3.2	38	1.5
Rude Health Chilled Organic Almond	0	0	1	53	0.3

How to Choose a Plant Based Milk

Which is the Best Milk For My Child?

I would choose a plant based milk that has high protein, fat, energy and is fortified with calcium and iodine. Top of my comparison table are Plenish organic unsweetened soya, Oatly Whole, Marks and Spencer's unsweetened soya.

While you might have seen others recommending The Mighty Pea Society pea mylk, this has excellent levels of calcium and protein, but does not contain iodine, and only a moderate energy content. Similarly, Rebel Kitchen has the highest energy, but contains no calcium or iodine, and is low protein.

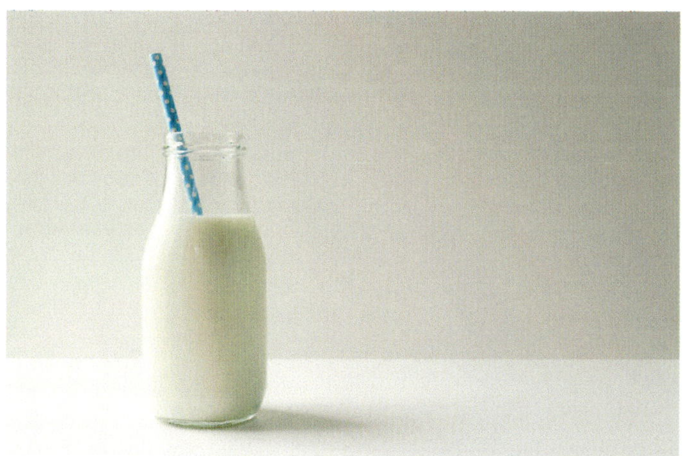

Postpartum and Beyond

EAT FOR HEALTH

Your Postpartum Body

Weight Loss After Giving Birth

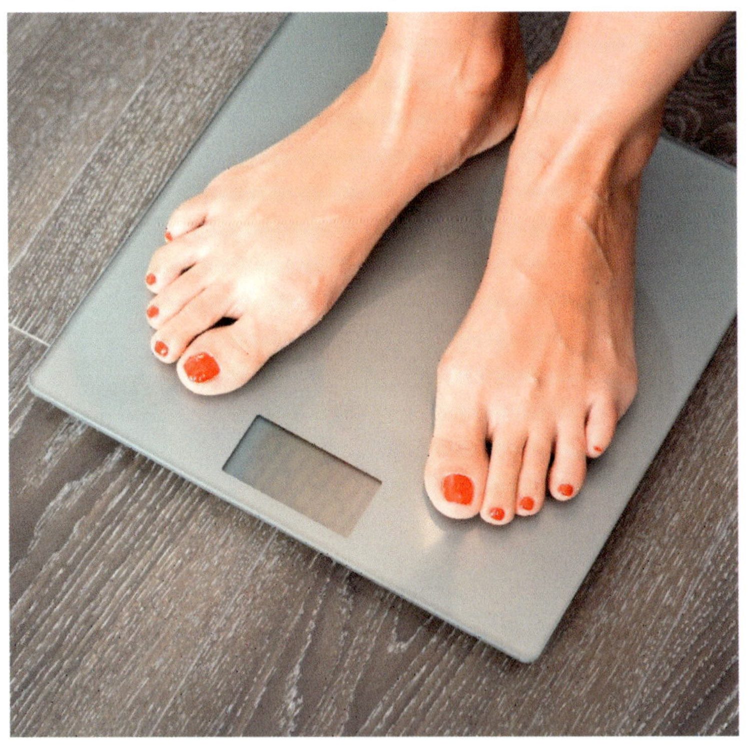

Postpartum and Beyond

EAT FOR HEALTH

Your Postpartum Body

Weight Loss After Giving Birth

While pregnancy and having a baby is one of the most exciting phases of life, it also brings about huge changes. One of those can be a physical change in appearance, after your body has gone through the incredible task of growing a human being and delivering them out to the world.

Having a new baby can be a huge psychological change, and coupled with feeling physically difficult many women can find that they feel different. I think women should be empowered to attain a healthy weight and feel good about themselves, including after having a baby. But I do think there shouldn't be societal pressure just to bounce back to your pre-pregnancy shape as soon as your baby has been born.

So what should you expect about your body shape and weight loss after giving birth? Firstly I think it's important to understand about the basis of the metabolic rate, weight gain and the role of gut microbiota.

Metabolism and Metabolic Rate

The word metabolism is often used interchangeably with basal metabolic rate, which is the number of calories you burn. Most people though when they think of metabolism, associate it with weight gain and weight loss.

Postpartum and Beyond

EAT FOR HEALTH

Your Postpartum Body

Metabolism and Burning Energy

Every day we metabolise our food, creating energy that we use in three different ways:

1. performing vital functions such as breathing to keep us alive.

2. thermogenesis: this is the process of digesting, absorbing and transporting the food you eat.

3. physical activity such as walking and exercise.

The basal metabolic rate (BMR) is the energy required for performing vital body functions at rest. Your brain, liver, heart and kidneys account for almost half of your BMR. An estimate of BMR can be calculated from your weight, age and gender.

Our BMR accounts for most of the energy we use, with thermogenesis only 10% and physical activity between 10-30%.

Metabolism and Weight

Many people assume that boosting your metabolism will help with weight gain, and that people who are overweight, have a slower metabolism.

In fact, people with a higher weight have a higher BMR and use more energy to perform everyday activities as it is harder to move about. Lean body mass (muscle) contributes most to your BMR, so the greater lean body mass you have, the higher your BMR.

Postpartum and Beyond

EAT FOR HEALTH

Your Postpartum Body

Managing Weight

Fundamentally what controls your weight is the balance of how much fuel you eat, compared with how much you consume. If you eat more than you need, you will store it as fat and gain weight. If you eat less than you need, you will lose weight. However, if you eat fewer calories than you need, this is sensed as starvation, and leads to a drop in BMR, meaning that you will lose less weight. But a slow gradual reduction in food intake, and weight loss, has less effect on reducing BMR.

Only in rare cases is the metabolic rate the reason for weight gain, for example with hypothyroid disease (under active thyroid). As most of us know, it is much easier to gain weight than lose it, and there are ideas that this is probably an evolutionary adaptation to protect us in times of famine, the so called 'thrifty gene hypothesis'.

However, using this hypothesis you might predict that everyone with freely available food would become obese, and this just isn't the case. So while a stable weight is partly due to energy balance, it appears it's more complicated.

Microbiota and Their Role in Metabolism

The gut microbiota contains trillions of single celled microorganisms, that play an important role in our health. Multiple associations between the gut microbiota and chemicals along metabolic pathways have been found, with suggestion that the gut microorganisms have a role in shaping metabolism.

Your Postpartum Body

Microbiota and Their Role in Metabolism...

Recent research has found that changing the composition of the microbiota, using prebiotic supplements (compounds that are not digestible by the human body, but preferentially nourish beneficial strains of gut microorganisms), is associated with improvement of some of the parameters of the metabolic syndrome (a name given to a set of conditions seen together including increased blood pressure, high blood sugar, a large waistline, and abnormal cholesterol or triglyceride levels).

In studies of special germ-free mice, who have no organisms living on or inside them, they found that faecal transplant from obese humans, was associated with a greater weight gain than mice that received microbes from healthy weight humans. This suggests that metabolic rate, and maintenance of a steady healthy weight, is more than the simple balance of energy in, equalling energy out.

Instead it is also impacted by your gut microbiota. Most studies of people that were obese have found that their gut microbiota is characterised by a narrower range of organisms (lower diversity). Long term weight gain (over 10 years) in humans is correlated with low microbiota diversity (narrow range of species of microorganisms), and this association is worsened by low dietary fibre intake.

How single celled microorganisms have such a profound effect on our weight and general health is astonishing, but it is probably mediated by a number of different routes.

Your Postpartum Body

Microbiota and Their Role in Metabolism...

Gut microbiota imbalance probably promotes weight gain and metabolic complications by a variety of mechanisms including immune dysregulation, altered energy regulation, altered gut hormone regulation, and proinflammatory mechanisms (such as lipopolysaccharide endotoxins crossing the gut barrier and entering the portal circulation).

Metabolic Rate Boosting Supplements

Dietary supplements are not required, unlike medicines, to prove that their products are safe or effective. Many of the items marketed as 'metabolic boosters' are ergogenic aids, meaning a performance enhancer that gives you a mental or physical improvement while exercising.

As discussed, exercise does increase your BMR but improved performance doesn't equate with further alteration of the BMR. Some items naturally found in our diet though have been found to alter performance, and caffeine is an example. Caffeine improves both aerobic and anaerobic performance and can marginally increase thermogenesis.

Postpartum and Beyond

EAT FOR HEALTH

Your Postpartum Body

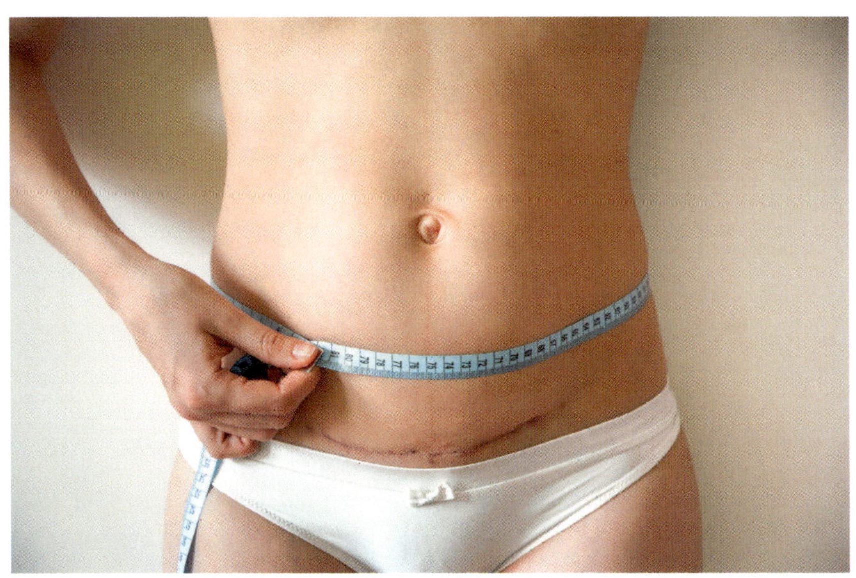

Postpartum and Beyond

EAT FOR HEALTH

Your Postpartum Body

Weight Gain After Birth

Gaining weight during pregnancy is completely normal. During pregnancy, as your body changes to enable your baby to grow, weight gain is partly made up of increased blood volume, placenta, uterus, amniotic fluid and of course your baby. Six weeks after birth, most women will lose half of the weight gained during pregnancy.

After six weeks, when thinking of weight loss, try to set realistic goals that are gradual and sustainable long term, rather than a crash diet with rapid weight loss and then rebound gain. Research has shown that the longer people can keep the weight off, the less likely they are to have rebound gain. Aim for approximately 0.5kg per week and focus on gradually increasing physical activity and making healthy choices.

If you are breastfeeding, your body will need approximately 500 extra calories per day but the exact amount depends on how often and how much your baby feeds. While some women find that weight loss is relatively easy while breastfeeding, others find that they start gaining weight, or can't lose their pregnancy weight until they wean. There are a number of possible reasons for this.

Firstly, you might not be eating enough. As discussed above, if you eat fewer calories than you need, this is sensed as starvation, and leads to a drop in BMR, meaning that you will lose less weight. While breastfeeding your body may be more sensitive to any drop in BMR and work to gaining weight and increase it. However, a slow gradual reduction in food intake, and weight loss, has less effect on reducing BMR.

Postpartum and Beyond

EAT FOR HEALTH

Your Postpartum Body

Weight Gain After Birth...

Instead of focusing on calorie restriction, think of making healthy choices instead, (see the beginning of the book), focusing on eating nutrient packed fruit, vegetables, whole grains, nuts, seeds, lean protein, and unsaturated fats.

Alternatively, you might be eating too much, and there can be a number of reasons why this might happen. The vast majority of new mums find that they are very sleep derived and it's easy to eat to try to obtain an energy boost when you are feeling exhausted. It's really easy to think that maternity leave and breastfeeding means you have a licence to eat as much cake as you fancy.

While I love cake too, breastfeeding won't mean that all your weight will just melt away, instead focus on making those healthy choices most of the time. Sometimes hunger is mistaken for thirst, and keeping hydrated is important while breastfeeding, so check you aren't thirsty first. Concentrate on eating mindfully because you are hungry.

You might be physically less active. Sometimes it is easy to mistake being busy with your children as physically active for example dashing between appointments or childcare in the car. Perhaps before you might have had a fast walk round the park, maybe now it's a stroll with your kids while they learn to walk or scoot.

Try to incorporate exercise into your routine when you are up to it and remember that every little counts, it doesn't have to be formalised exercise in a gym.

Postpartum and Beyond

EAT FOR HEALTH

Your Postpartum Body

Weight Gain After Birth...

I think most new parents would say that while having a baby can bring immense joy, it is also stressful. Worries about birth, then feeding, looking after your baby, guessing the meaning of their cries, the new found responsibility, and the sleep deprivation can all have an effect on your eating pattern. Faced with stress, some people eat less, while for others they eat more. Acute stress is more likely to induce undereating, while chronic stress is more likely to induce overeating.

Glucocorticoid hormones, the effector molecules of the stress response, have been found to increase the tendency to eat high-calorie, palatable foods. Find ways to reduce stress by improving your sleep if possible, having a quiet walk, doing some gentle exercise like yoga, doing some meditation, have a relaxing bath, or find something that works for you and find the time for it.

Summary

Your basal metabolic rate is determined by your genes and your body composition. Exercise can increase your metabolic rate and is important for so many factors of general health. While maintaining a steady weight used to be thought of in terms of simple energy balance, evidence of the important role of the gut microbiota, might explain why some people can appear to eat much more than the energy they expend, without gaining weight.

Your Postpartum Body

Summary...

Ultimately the best way to support your metabolism, metabolic rate and a healthy weight is by regular exercise (see the following section) and a healthy diet that follows these principles:

- eat lots of different coloured fruit and vegetables
- choose whole grains (bulgur wheat, millet, sweet potatoes, brown rice, brown bread)
- eat a handful of nuts a day and add seeds to your food
- drink water
- eat oily fish twice a week
- chose lean or plant based protein
- enjoy healthy unsaturated fats such avocados, rapeseed and extra virgin olive oils.
- support your microbiota to flourish by eating fermented foods, kefir, and 30g of fibre a day.

When is it Safe to Start Exercising Again?

Exercise is really important for health in general and bone health. Current guidance is to aim to walk, cycle, run, play tennis, Pilates or another sport for at least 30 minutes five times a week. Only consider this when you feel physically recovered from giving birth, and gradually introduce it back into your routine where possible.

You might find it initially impossible, but as a mother, once my children were walking, I found that I spent most of the day running around chasing after them! Before they were mobile, carrying, lifting, pushing them in a pram is all still exercise too. All exercise counts, you don't have to be in your gym clothes, and it doesn't have to be formal.

If you had an uncomplicated vaginal delivery and you feel well, you can start gentle exercise such as walking, pelvic floor exercises and gentle stretches as soon as you feel up to it. It's still a good idea to wait until after you have had a postnatal check (approximately 6 weeks after delivery) before you start any high-impact exercise such as running or other aerobic sports.

If you had a c-section, your doctor may recommend that you wait for at least 12 weeks before starting any high-impact exercise again. However you gave birth, you should avoid swimming until 7 days after your postnatal bleeding has stopped.

During pregnancy, your ligaments become more flexible, as this allows your pelvis to widen in preparation for birth. This doesn't change straight away after giving birth and can take a few months to return to normal. Therefore, you are at an increased risk of soft tissue injury. Your core and abdominal muscles will also probably be weaker than they used to be.

When is it Safe to Start Exercising Again?...

Pelvic floor exercises are just as important as while you were pregnant. Your pelvic floor muscles take a huge strain while you are pregnant and during birth. If they are weak you might notice that you leak urine when you cough or sneeze (stress incontinence). It's a good idea to get them strong again by continuing pelvic floor exercises when you feel up to it.

Exercise not only has an important role in physical health, but has also been shown to reduce postnatal depression (PND). In a meta-analysis where 52 studies were combined (totalling over 131,000 participants), they found that prenatal exercise reduced the risk of getting PND and also the severity. Another smaller meta-analysis found that postnatal exercise also reduced depressive symptoms.

Exercise in Children

Current guidance in the UK is for children under the age of 5 years old to have 3 hours of exercise a day. This can come from a range of activities and doesn't have to be inside. Exercise improves sleep, develops muscles and bones, maintains health and weight, contributes to brain development, encourages movement and co-ordination and builds social skills and relationships. For babies start with tummy time, reaching, pulling, rolling etc.

Children aged 1-4 years old the 3 hours of exercise a day can be anything, for example playing, cycling, scooting, running, skipping, hopping, swimming, catching a ball, jumping, or messy play. Between 3-4 years old, at least 1 hour out of the 3, should include moderate to vigorous activity where they get a little out of breath and sweaty.

Between 5-18 years this drops to a minimum of 1 hour of physical activity a day, including both aerobic activities and strength or resistance training.

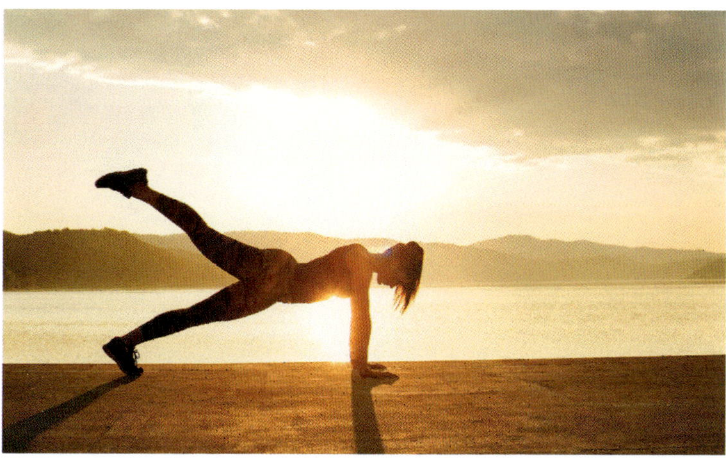

Close

I hope that I've answered all your questions about what to eat during breastfeeding and beyond, and you find this guide both useful and reassuring. I'd love to hear how you get on. Send me a message on Instagram at @healthyeatingdr or email me at info@healthyeatingdr.com

To help guide you with this information, try using my breastfeeding meal planner and nutrient checklist (also available to download from the Free Resources section of my website https://healthyeatingdr.com/what-nutrition-is-needed-during-breastfeeding/).

If you would like more information about science backed nutrition, check out my video courses available through my website.

Next time you get pregnant, check out my meal planner and nutrient checklist for pregnancy, available on the Free Resources section of my website.

Once again, congratulations on the birth of your baby and I hope all goes very smoothly for you.

Postpartum and Beyond

EAT FOR HEALTH

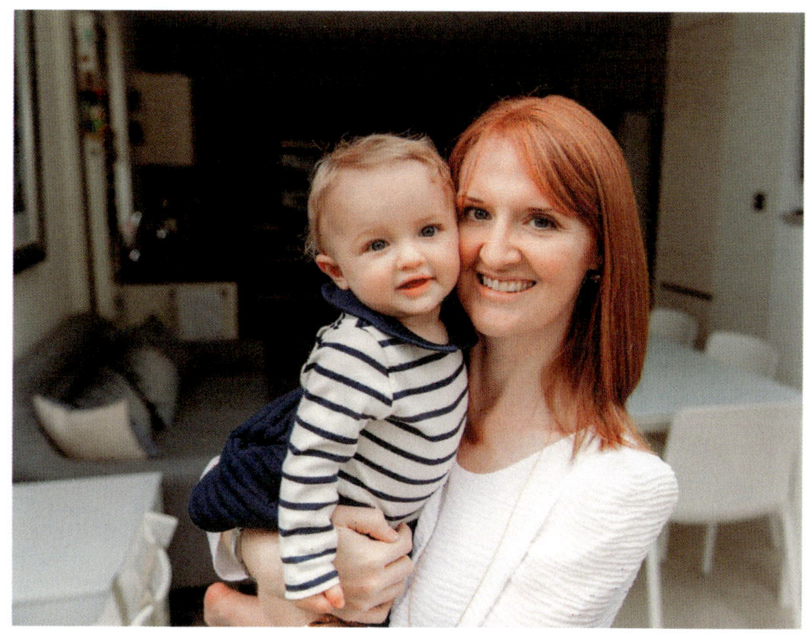

HEALTHY EATING DR

fact not fiction

I'm delighted you downloaded my fridge planner and nutrient checklist to use while you are breastfeeding.

I created this planner and check list to help give you a general frame work for nutritional needs. I know how difficult it can be adjusting to motherhood, and wanted to lighten the burden of yet another thing to remember for new mums. Many women find this a challenging time, and eating healthily might not be top of your list of priorities. So the checklist was designed to help remind and guide you.

The Planner

How you use the planner is entirely up to you, but I suggest writing out the name of your meals for the week, adding items you need to the shopping list, enabling you to be more organised. I recommend that you consider batch cooking, which can help reduce the pressure of daily cooking and food preparation.

The Checklist

On page 3 is the meal planner and checklist combined. I'd suggest ticking off the checklist through the day to ensure that you are supporting your nutrient needs. If you would rather a simpler version without the planner, use page 4 as a weekly check instead. Page 4 has foods rich in micronutrients needed in greater quantities while breastfeeding, such as calcium, selenium, iodine and vitamin D. While you are breast feeding women and your periods have not restarted, you need less iron than usual, so this is not included on the checklist. To make it as easy as possible, I've used average portion sizes so there shouldn't be any need to weigh your food.

Dr Harriet Holme MA Hons Cantab MBBS PhD RNutr
@healthyeatingdr
www.healthyeatingdr.com

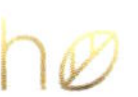

HEALTHY EATING DR

fact not fiction

How to Use

I recommend that you print this document A4 size, and then stick it to your fridge or noticeboard. For greater sustainability you could laminate or pop it in a poly pocket and wipe clean after use.

I created this planner and check list to help give you a general frame work for nutritional needs. However, this can't take the place of personalised nutrition advice, tailored to your individual health needs. If you have any specific health concerns or food allergies, you could take this along to discuss with your health care provider.

About Me

Hi I'm Dr Harriet Holme, a Registered Nutritionist, specialising in nutrition science and evidence based nutrition. I studied medicine at the University of Cambridge and worked for over a decade as a paediatric doctor in the NHS. I completed a PhD in genetics from University College London before becoming a Registered Nutritionist with the Association of Nutrition. I now use these uniquely developed skills for the benefit of my clients and students, consulting as a Registered Nutritionist and lecturing in culinary science and nutrition.

Dr Harriet Holme MA Hons Cantab MBBS PhD RNutr
@healthyeatingdr
www.healthyeatingdr.com

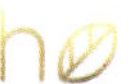

HEALTHY EATING DR

fact not fiction

breastfeeding mothers

	Monday	Tuesday	Wednesday	Thursday	Friday	Saturday	Sunday	Shopping List
Breakfast								
Lunch								
Dinner								
5 fruit/veg	☐	☐	☐	☐	☐	☐	☐	
30g nuts	☐	☐	☐	☐	☐	☐	☐	
30g fibre	☐	☐	☐	☐	☐	☐	☐	
2-3 portions/ wk oily fish	☐	☐	☐	☐	☐	☐	☐	
1250mg calcium	☐	☐	☐	☐	☐	☐	☐	
10mcg vitamin D	☐	☐	☐	☐	☐	☐	☐	
70mcg selenium	☐	☐	☐	☐	☐	☐	☐	
200mcg iodine	☐	☐	☐	☐	☐	☐	☐	

Dr Harriet Holme MA Hons Cantab MBBS PhD RNutr
@healthyeatingdr
www.healthyeatingdr.com

Calcium

To ensure you are eating 1250mg of calcium a day include these calcium rich foods:

- 100ml cow's milk (1/2 cup) ~ 125mg
- 100ml fortified oat milk ~120mg
- 100ml fortified nut milks ~120mg
- 100ml The Mighty pea mylk ~186mg
- 100ml fortified coconut milk ~120mg
- matchbox size piece of cheese ~220mg
- 120mg yoghurt ~200mg
- 100mls (/2 cup) fortified orange juice ~120mg
- 1 slice calcium fortified bread ~190mg
- 1/2 tin sardines (with bones) ~260mg
- 50g (small portion) whitebait ~430mg
- 6 pieces of scampi (90g) ~190mg
- 2 slices wholemeal bread ~54mg
- 2 slices white bread ~100mg
- 1 pitta bread ~60mg
- 1 medium orange ~75mg
- 85mg boiled broccoli (2 spears) ~34mg
- 75mg spring greens ~55mg

Vitamin D

To ensure you are eating 10mcg vitamin D a day include these foods or consider taking a supplement:

- 100g salmon ~10-18mcg
- 100g canned tuna ~5-6mcg
- 250mls (1 cup) whole cow's milk ~3mcg
- 1 egg ~1mcg

Selenium

To ensure you are eating 70mcg selenium a day include these selenium rich foods:

- 1 brazil nut ~50-80mcg
- 100g crab ~130mcg
- 100mg mussels ~65mcg
- 100g mackerel ~35mcg
- 100g cod ~ 26mcg
- 30g cashew nuts ~8mcg

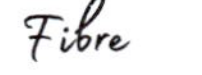

Fibre

To ensure you are eating 30g fibre a day include these fibre rich foods:

- 2 slices wholemeal bread ~5g
- 150g wholemeal spaghetti ~5g
- 50g porridge ~5g
- medium baked potato ~5g
- 80g raspberries ~2.5g
- apple ~2g
- banana 2g
- 100g (3 spears) broccoli boiled~2.3g
- 100g boiled carrots ~2.5g
- 30g almonds ~2g
- 100g chickpeas ~4-5g
- 100g boiled peas ~4.5g
- 80g baked beans (in tomato sauce) ~3g

Dr Harriet Holme MA Hons Cantab MBBS PhD RNutr
@healthyeatingdr
www.healthyeatingdr.com

Iodine

To ensure you are eating 200mcg iodine a day include these iodine rich foods:

- 200ml cow's milk ~50-100mcg
- 200ml organic cow's milk ~30-60mcg
- 150mg Yoghurt ~50-100mcg
- 40g cheese ~15mcg
- 120mg haddock ~390mcg
- 120mg cod ~230mcg
- 120mg plaice ~27mcg
- 120g salmon fillet ~17mcg
- 100g canned tuna ~12mcg
- 120g prawns ~12mcg
- 170g scampi ~160mcg
- 1 egg ~25mcg
- 100g meat / poultry ~10mcg
- 30g nuts ~6mcg
- 1 slice of bread ~ 5mcg
- 1 portion fruit or vegetables ~3mcg

References

https://www.bda.uk.com/resource/calcium.html

https://ods.od.nih.gov/factsheets/VitaminD-HealthProfessional/

https://assets.publishing.service.gov.uk/government/uploads/system/uploads/attachment_data/file/339431/SACN_Selenium_and_Health_2013.pdf

https://www.bda.uk.com/resource/iodine.html

https://www.nutrition.org.uk/healthyliving/basics/fibre.html

https://www.nhs.uk/live-well/eat-well/how-to-get-more-fibre-into-your-diet/

https://www.bda.uk.com/resource/fibre.html

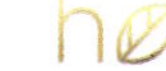

Postpartum and Beyond

EAT FOR HEALTH

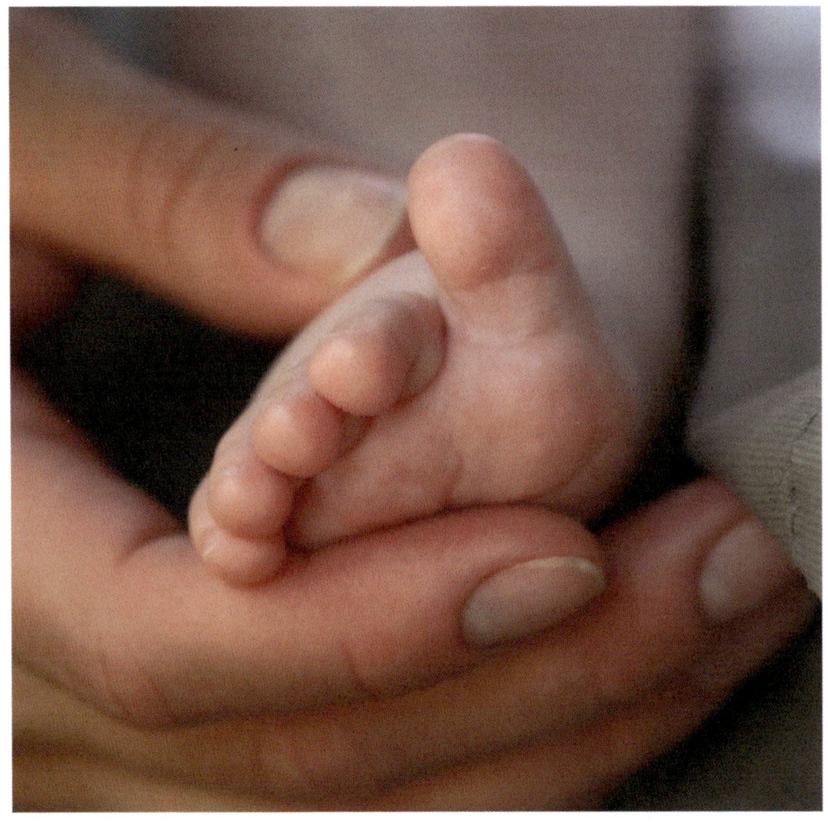

Printed in Great Britain
by Amazon